Local Anaesthesia in Dentistry

Local Anaesthesia in Dentistry

J.A. Baart
H.S. Brand
(Editors)

Translated by
Joanne Orton, Henk Brand and Jacques Baart

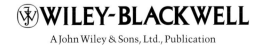

A John Wiley & Sons, Ltd., Publication

This edition first published 2009
© 2009 Blackwell Publishing Ltd
© 2006 Bohn Stafleu van Loghum, Houten

This edition of Lokale anesthesie in de tandheelkunde/Local anaesthesia in dentistry, edited by J.A. Baart and H.S. Brand is published by arrangement with *Bohn Stafleu van Loghum BV, Het Spoor 2, Postbus 246, 3990 GA Houten, The Netherlands.*

Translation of this edition undertaken by Blackwell Publishing Ltd.

Blackwell Publishing was acquired by John Wiley & Sons in February 2007. Blackwell's publishing programme has been merged with Wiley's global Scientific, Technical, and Medical business to form Wiley-Blackwell.

Registered office
John Wiley & Sons Ltd, The Atrium, Southern Gate, Chichester, West Sussex, PO19 8SQ, United Kingdom

Editorial offices
9600 Garsington Road, Oxford, OX4 2DQ, United Kingdom
2121 State Avenue, Ames, Iowa 50014-8300, USA

For details of our global editorial offices, for customer services and for information about how to apply for permission to reuse the copyright material in this book please see our website at www.wiley.com/wiley-blackwell.

Library of Congress Cataloging-in-Publication Data

Lokale anesthesie in de tandheelkunde. English.
    Local anaesthesia in dentistry / [edited by] J.A. Baart, H.S. Brand.
        p. ; cm.
    Originally published in Dutch: Lokale anesthesie in de tandheelkunde / J.A. Baart, H.S. Brand (redactie). 2006.
        Includes bibliographical references and index.
        ISBN 978-1-4051-8436-6 (pbk. : alk. paper)
    1. Anesthesia in dentistry.   2. Local anesthesia.   I. Baart, J.A. (Jacobus Andries), 1950–   II. Brand, H.S.   III. Title.
        [DNLM: 1. Anesthesia, Dental.   2. Anesthesia, Local. WO 460 L863 2008a]

    RK510.L6513 2008
    617.9′676–dc22

                                                                          2008013077

A catalogue record for this book is available from the British Library.

Lokale anesthesie in de tandheelkunde ISBN 9031340936

Set in 8.5/12 Utopia by Graphicraft Limited, Hong Kong
Printed in Singapore by Fabulous Printers Pte Ltd

1   2009
Illustrated by P. Brugman, A.A. van Horssen and M. Kunen

Contents

Foreword

The significance of local anaesthesia in the world of dentistry can hardly be underestimated. Local anaesthesia ensures, for one thing, that dental treatment may be a comfortable and painless experience for the patient. It also enables the dentist to carry out the treatment in a calm and concentrated manner.

The use of local anaesthesia in dentistry for adults and children requires a thorough knowledge of anatomy, pharmacology and the manner in which the anaesthetic must be administered. Besides this, of course, it is also necessary to possess knowledge of the local and systemic complications and of the use of local anaesthesia in so-called patients 'at risk'. This book deals extensively with all these topics, as well as legal aspects.

Local Anaesthesia in Dentistry is aimed mainly at dentists and dental students. The book will also be of service to those training to be a dental or medical specialist. The editors, J.A. Baart and H.S. Brand, must be complimented for the design of the book and for the collaboration they secured from the authors, all experts in this subject. They have succeeded in providing the reader with the necessary information in a balanced way. Indeed, it is an easy-to-read and clearly illustrated manual.

Finally, the publishers deserve recognition for the handsome layout.

Amsterdam, Summer 2008
Prof. Dr I. van der Waal

Editors and authors

Editors

J.A. Baart, Academic Centre for Dentistry Amsterdam/Vrije Universiteit Medical Centre, Department of Oral and Maxillofacial Surgery, Amsterdam, The Netherlands.

H.S. Brand, Academic Centre for Dentistry Amsterdam, Department of Oral and Maxillofacial Surgery and Department of Basic Dental Sciences, Amsterdam, The Netherlands.

Authors

H.P. van den Akker, Academic Centre for Dentistry Amsterdam/Academic Medical Centre, Department of Oral and Maxillofacial Surgery, Amsterdam, The Netherlands.

L.H.D.J. Booij, Radboud University Medical Centre Nijmegen, Department of Anaesthesiology, Nijmegen, The Netherlands.

J.F.L. Bosgra, Academic Centre for Dentistry Amsterdam/Vrije Universiteit Medical Centre, Department of Oral and Maxillofacial Surgery, Amsterdam, The Netherlands.

W.G. Brands, General Dental Practitioner/Part-time Judge, Civil Section, Court of Utrecht, The Netherlands/Radboud University Medical Centre Nijmegen, Department of Social and Preventive Dentistry, Nijmegen, The Netherlands.

T.M.G.J. van Eijden†, Academic Centre for Dentistry Amsterdam, Department of Functional Anatomy, Amsterdam, The Netherlands.

J.F.M. Fennis, Radboud University Medical Centre Nijmegen, Department of General Internal Medicine, Nijmegen, The Netherlands.

F.W.A. Frankenmolen, Paediatric Dental Centre, Beuningen, The Netherlands.

A.L. Frankhuijzen, Vrije Universiteit Medical Centre, Department of Pharmacology, Amsterdam, The Netherlands.

G.E.J. Langenbach, Academic Centre for Dentistry Amsterdam, Department of Functional Anatomy, Amsterdam, The Netherlands.

Dedication

Dedicated to the memory of Theo van Eijden (1951–2007)
– researcher, teacher and friend.

Introduction: a short history of local anaesthesia

J.A. Baart and J.F.L. Bosgra

General anaesthesia already existed before local anaesthesia became available. Actually, general anaesthesia was introduced by the American dentist Horace Wells. In 1844, together with his wife Elizabeth, he witnessed a demonstration whereby the circus owner Colton intoxicated a number of volunteers with laughing gas. One of the volunteers hit himself hard on a chair but did not even grimace. Horace Wells noticed this and concluded that a patient, having inhaled laughing gas, might be able to undergo an extraction without pain. A few days later Wells took the experiment upon himself and asked a colleague to extract one of his molars after he had inhaled some laughing gas. It was a success. Wells independently organised some additional extraction sessions, after which the Massachusetts General Hospital invited him for a demonstration. This demonstration turned out to be a fiasco. The patient was insufficiently anaesthetised since not enough laughing gas was administered. Wells' life, which had initially been so successful, became a disaster. The physician Morton, a previous assistant to Wells, absconded with the idea of general anaesthesia, but used ether instead of laughing gas for a 'painless sleep'. Morton denied in every possible way that he had stolen the idea from Wells. Wells was greatly incensed by this. Furthermore, Wells was no longer able to practise as a dentist. He became a tradesman of canaries and domestic products and became addicted to sniffing ether. Eventually he was imprisoned for throwing sulphuric acid over some ladies of easy virtue. At the age of 33 years he made an end to his life in prison by cutting his femoral artery.

The discovery of local anaesthesia is a very different story. One of the first to gain experience with this form of anaesthesia was Sigmund Freud, in 1884. Freud experimented with the use of cocaine. Cocaine had been used for several centuries by the Incas in Peru to increase their stamina. Freud used cocaine in the treatment of some of his patients, and then became addicted himself. The German surgeon August Bier observed a demonstration in 1891, whereby the internist Quincke injected – for diagnostic purposes – a cocaine solution into a patient's epidural area, thus anaesthetising and paralysing the legs. Bier took this discovery to his clinic in Kiel and decided to try the technique first on himself and only thereafter to operate on patients under local anaesthesia. Together with his colleague, senior doctor Hildebrandt, he decided to perform an experiment. Bier volunteered to be the guinea pig and Hildebrandt administered a spinal injection to his boss. This failed, however, due to the fact that the syringe containing the cocaine solution did not fit the needle so a lot of liquor leaked through the needle. It was then Hildebrandt's turn as the test subject and Bier succeeded in administering an epidural anaesthesia with a cocaine solution. After a few minutes Hildebrandt reported that his leg muscles were numb and his legs were tingling. Bier tested the efficacy of the local anaesthesia by sticking a large injection needle deep into Hildebrandt's upper leg. Hildebrandt did not feel a thing, even when Bier hit his femur skin hard with a wooden hammer. After 45 minutes the local anaesthetic began to wear off. The gentlemen then went out for dinner and enjoyed cognacs and good cigars. The next morning, however, the local and systemic disadvantages of this local anaesthesia came to light. Bier had a raging headache after his failed anaesthetic, which lasted one week and would only go away if he lay down. Nevertheless he continued to operate. Hildebrandt was in worse shape. The next day he called in sick; he felt dizzy and was vomiting continually. Walking was difficult, partly because of haemorrhages in his upper and lower leg. On the basis of all these disadvantages Bier concluded that he would refrain from treating his patients under local anaesthesia. Later Bier strayed from regular medicine and became an alternative medicine fanatic. However, Bier's extensive observations and descriptions of his experiments with local anaesthesia did not go unnoticed.

In 1899, the French surgeon Tuffer was unaware of Bier's work but operated on a young lady with a hip sarcoma under local anaesthesia, applying a cocaine solution to the spinal canal. Several years later he operated on patients under local anaesthesia in the kidney, stomach and even the thoracic wall. The first use of local anaesthesia in dentistry is attributed to the American Halsted, who anaesthetised himself with a cocaine solution.

Because of the high toxicity and addictive effects of cocaine, a safer local anaesthetic was sought. This was eventually found in 1905 in the form of procaine, an ester derivative of cocaine. Procaine became known under the brand name of Novocaine ('the new cocaine'). This remedy was used for many years, but after a while a stronger anaesthetic was needed. During the Second World War the Swedish scientist Nils Lofgren succeeded in making the amide compound lidocaine. Lidocaine remedy works faster and more effectively than cocaine and is not addictive. However, how to administer the local anaesthetic remained a problem. In 1947, the American company Novocol marketed the cartridge syringe, glass cartridges with local anaesthetic and disposable needles. With this, modern local anaesthesia was born. Lidocaine and articaine, which was introduced in the 1970s, are now the most commonly used local anaesthetics in dentistry.

Further reading

Bennion, E. (1986) *Antique Dental Instruments.* Sotheby's Publications, London.

Richards, J.M. (1977) *Who Is Who in Architecture, from 1400 to the Present Day.* Weidefeld and Nicolson, London.

Sydow, F.-W. (1987) Geschichte der Lokal- und Leitungsanaesthesie. In: Zinganell, K. (ed.) *Anaesthesie – historisch gesehen.* Springer, Berlin/Heidelberg.

1 Pain and impulse conduction

L.H.D.J. Booij

According to the World Health Organisation pain is defined as an 'unpleasant sensation that occurs from imminent tissue damage'. From a physiological perspective, pain is a warning system. During dental treatment, patients will experience pain as something unpleasant.

1.1 Pain receptors

Pain stimuli are primarily generated by the relatively amorph sensory nerve endings of the Aδ and C fibres. These free nerve endings (nociceptors; see Figure 1.1) are sensitive to a variety of mechanical, thermal and chemical stimuli and are therefore called polymodal. Nociceptors do not display adaptation: nociceptive responses will occur as long as the stimulus is present. Nociceptors have a high threshold for activation. The detection of the stimulus is performed by the receptors, present on the sensory nerve endings, that convert the stimulus into an electric signal. This process is called transduction.

During tissue damage, several substances are released that are able to stimulate the nociceptors, such as histamine, serotonin, bradykinin, prostaglandin E_2 and interleukins. These substances activate the nociceptors and reduce their threshold (sensitisation).

Nociceptors are also present in the teeth and the oral cavity and are usually sensitive to a specific neurotransmitter. Most nerve fibres, however, contain various nociceptors.

The sensory nervous system also contains 'physiological' sensors. These are small end organs of the sensory nerves, such as the Krause, Meisner and Pacini bodies (see Figure 1.2). These 'physiological' sensors usually only respond to one specific stimulus (warmth, touch, smell, etc.) and are, as such, unimodal. Besides this, they exhibit the phenomenon of adaptation; the response to stimulus disappears during prolonged or persistent stimulation. In the case of excessive stimulation, these 'physiological' sensors may also initiate pain sensation.

Figure 1.1
Nociceptors.

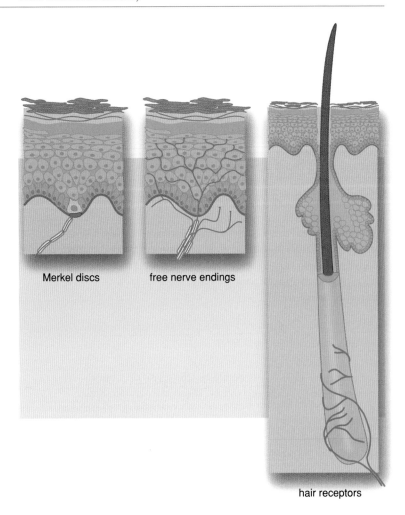

Merkel discs   free nerve endings

hair receptors

Figure 1.2
Physiological sensors.

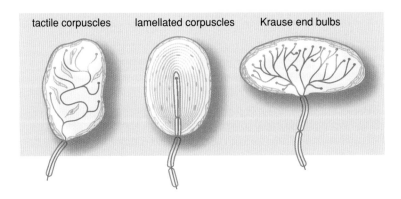

tactile corpuscles   lamellated corpuscles   Krause end bulbs

1.2   Nerve impulse transmission

The stimuli, received by the nociceptors and converted into nerve impulses, eventually must be interpreted in the brain. The nerve impulse is transported within the sensory nervous system, wherein three nerve fibres are successively linked. The first nerve fibres form the peripheral nerve. The second and third are present in the central nervous system and form nerve bundles (pathways or tracts). The cell nuclei of the individual neurons are grouped together in ganglia and nuclei.

1.2.1   The structure of the peripheral nerve

Nociceptive stimuli are transported along sensory thinly myelinated Aδ and unmyelinated C fibres. Other types of nerve fibres are involved in the transport of other sensory stimuli (see Box 1.1).

A peripheral nerve is composed of nerve fibres from a group of neurons, enwrapped in a connective tissue network. The individual fibres may, or may not be, surrounded by an isolating myelin layer, Schwann's sheath. The cell body is the metabolic centre of the neuron (Figure 1.3) where most cell organelles are produced. Dendrites transport impulses towards the cell body and axons transmit signals away from the cell body. Some axons are surrounded by a myelin sheath, others are not. The axons and dendrites are elongated and form the nerve fibres. At the end of the dendrites, receptors are present that can receive signals. At the end of

---

Box 1.1 Nociceptive pathways

In the body, nociceptive stimuli are received by nociceptors and then propagated via an Aδ or C fibre. The first are thinly myelinated with a fast transmission of stimuli, whereas the second are unmyelinated with a slow transmission.

The C fibres conduct impulses generated by temperature, pain and itching. The Aα fibres conduct motor impulses for the body's posture and movement; the Aβ fibres transport impulses generated by touch and signals from the skin mechano-receptors; and the Aδ fibres conduct pain impulses, temperature signals and signals to maintain the muscular tone.

The cell bodies of these primary neurons are located in the dorsal root ganglion. The axons run through Lissauer's tract to the dorsal horn of the spinal cord, where they connect to the secondary sensory neuron in Rexed's laminae. This secondary sensory neuron crosses the midline and ascends as the spinothalamic tract. The spinothalamic tract forms synapses with nuclei of the thalamus, where it projects onto the somatosensory cortex. Descending pathways from the somatosensory cortex modulate the nociceptive system. From these fibres, the neurotransmitters serotonin and noradrenalin are released.

Figure B1.1
Primary afferent axons.

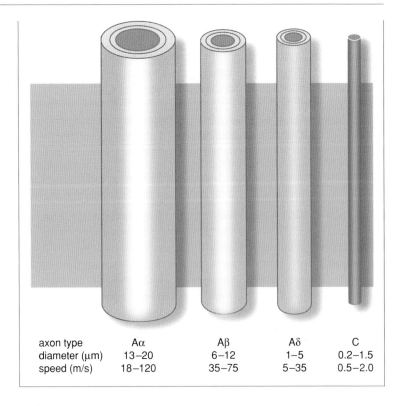

Figure B1.1
Primary afferent axons.

axon type	Aα	Aβ	Aδ	C
diameter (μm)	13–20	6–12	1–5	0.2–1.5
speed (m/s)	18–120	35–75	5–35	0.5–2.0

the axons are synapses, where the impulse is transmitted to another nerve cell or to a cell of the end organ.

Nerves are bundles of nerve fibres held together by connective tissue (Figure 1.4). Each individual axon is surrounded by connective tissue (endoneurium). Bundles of nerve fibres form a fascicle, which is also held together by connective tissue (perineurium). A number of fascicles are held together again by connective tissue (epineurium), forming a nerve.

1.2.2   Impulse formation

The generation and conduction of impulses in nerve fibres is a complicated process. In order to excite electrical impulses, a change in electrical charge must take place. Cells are surrounded by a semipermeable membrane that is only permeable to water. A selective ion pump actively pumps potassium ions into the cell and sodium ions out of the cell. This results in a concentration gradient of sodium and potassium ions over the membrane. The cell cytoplasm contains a high concentration of negatively charged proteins, which give the cell a negative charge compared with its environment. Extracellularly, negatively charged ions are also present, primarily chloride ions. On both sides of the membrane, the electrical charge is balanced by positively charged ions (sodium, potassium, calcium). Because the concentration of anions on the inside is

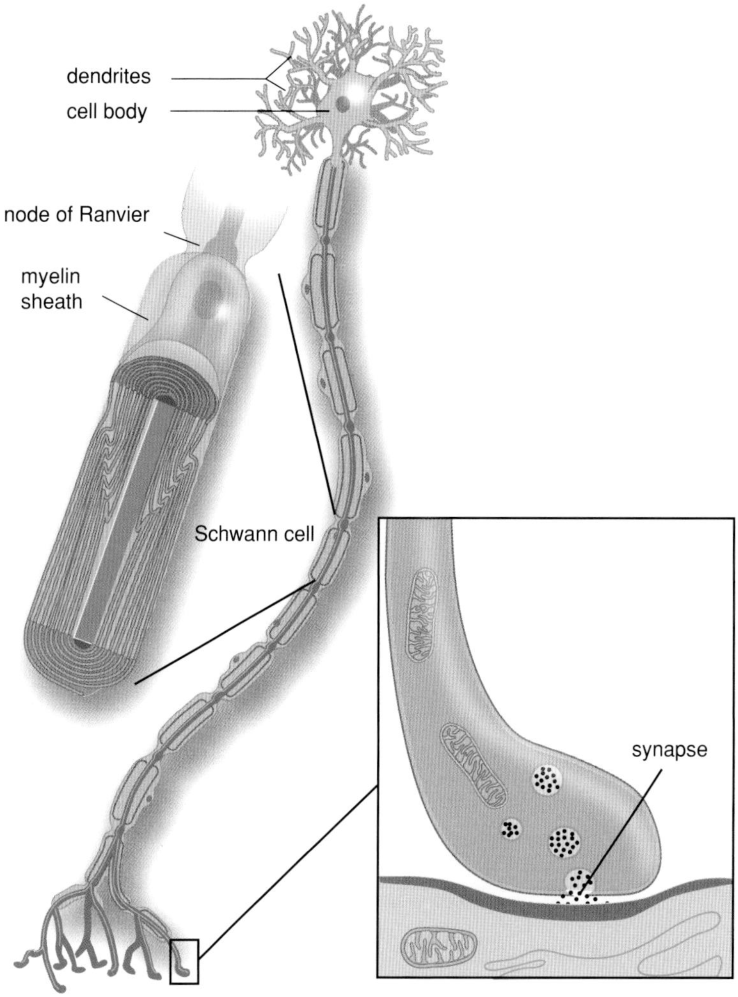

Figure 1.3
The nerve cell.

dendrites

cell body

node of Ranvier

myelin sheath

Schwann cell

synapse

slightly higher than on the outside, the number of cations inside will therefore be higher than outside. This causes a transmembrane potential difference of −60 mV, called the resting potential.

The membrane contains ion channels with an open and closed state (Figure 1.5). These channels can be activated by an electrical stimulus ('voltage-gated') or by a chemical stimulus ('ligand-gated') (see Box 1.2). When ion channels are open, ions move along the concentration gradient. At rest, primarily potassium channels are open, so that potassium ions try to leave the cell. However, the relative overload of anions in the cell (proteins) counteracts the outflow of cations. When the sodium channels of the membrane open, sodium ions will move in: in other words, the membrane has a hole.

The inflow of sodium ions distorts the electrical equilibrium, so that a local depolarisation occurs and potassium ions can leave the cell. This

Figure 1.4
The peripheral nerve.

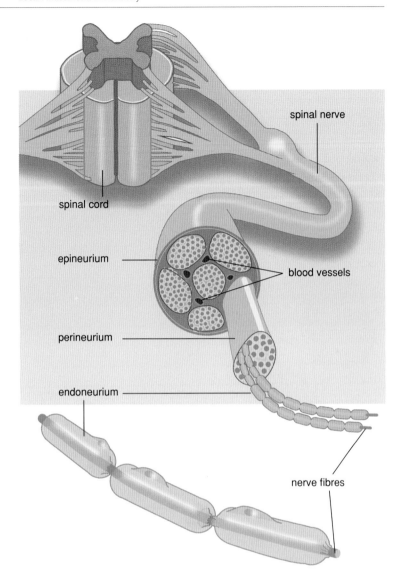

spinal nerve

spinal cord

epineurium

blood vessels

perineurium

endoneurium

nerve fibres

restores the balance between anions and cations (repolarisation). During depolarisation and the beginning of repolarisation, no new depolarisation can occur (refractory period).

When the local depolarisation is slight, the equilibrium is quickly restored (Figure 1.6). Only when the local depolarisation reaches a certain threshold value (approx. −50 mV), does an action potential appear. Thus there is an 'all-or-none' effect.

The height of the threshold value, necessary for an action potential to develop, is determined by several factors, such as the duration and strength of the depolarising stimulus and the status of the receptor. Through this, the voltage-gated sodium channels are opened, so that an influx of sodium occurs and the membrane polarity reverses.

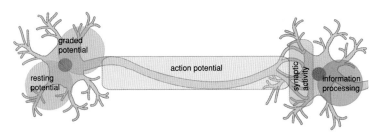

Figure 1.5
Semi-permeable membrane
with ion channels.

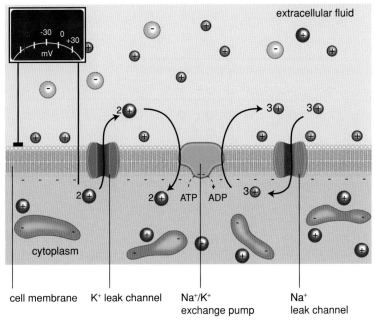

extracellular fluid

cytoplasm

cell membrane   K⁺ leak channel   Na⁺/K⁺
                                         exchange pump

Na⁺
leak channel

- Cl⁻

+ K⁺

+ Na⁺

Box 1.2

Ion channels are of great importance for the generation, conduction and transfer of nerve impulses. Activation of these receptors may occur by an electrical stimulus (voltage-gated channels) or by a neurotransmitter (ligand-gated channels). Once activated the channel opens, which allows the passage of ions, causing a depolarisation of the cell membrane.

Voltage-gated ion channels are, amongst others, the fast sodium channels and calcium channels involved in impulse formation in the heart and in impulse conduction in the nerve fibres. Examples of ligand-gated ion channels are acetylcholine receptors, glutamate receptors and GABA receptors.

Figure B1.2 A–C

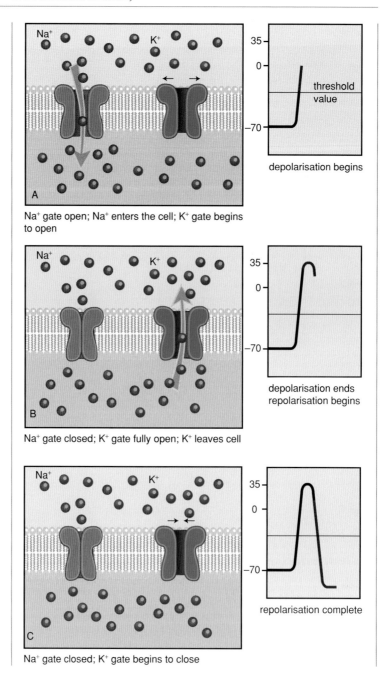

A

Na⁺ gate open; Na⁺ enters the cell; K⁺ gate begins to open

depolarisation begins

B

Na⁺ gate closed; K⁺ gate fully open; K⁺ leaves cell

depolarisation ends
repolarisation begins

C

Na⁺ gate closed; K⁺ gate begins to close

repolarisation complete

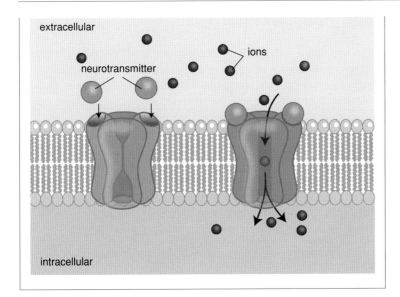

Figure B1.2 D
Activation of a ligand-gated ion channel.

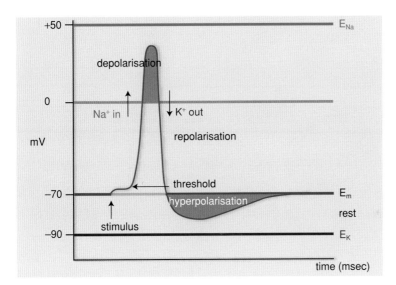

Figure 1.6
The action potential.

The sodium channels remain open only for approx. 1 millisecond, after which they close again. The potassium channels are then still open, and the outflow of potassium through voltage-gated potassium channels restores the electrical equilibrium, and even hyperpolarisation takes place. Then the voltage-gated potassium channels close and the sodium–potassium pump restores the starting situation. The number of sodium and potassium ions that has to be moved in order to generate an action potential is only very small.

1.2.3   Impulse conduction and transfer

Once a stimulus is converted into an action potential, the action potential must be propagated along the nerve. This occurs through sequential depolarisations along the membrane, which are initiated by the activation of fast sodium channels. In myelinated nerves, sodium channels are only present at the gaps in the myelin sheath, the nodes of Ranvier, which causes a jumping (saltatory) conduction (Figure 1.7A). In unmyelinated nerve fibres, the conduction is a continuous process (Figure 1.7B).

Because the sensory nervous system consists of three successive neurons, the stimulus must be transferred from one nerve cell to another. This transmission is conducted by neurotransmitters in synapses. The neurotransmitter is released presynaptically and activates postsynaptic

Figure 1.7 A

Saltatory conduction.

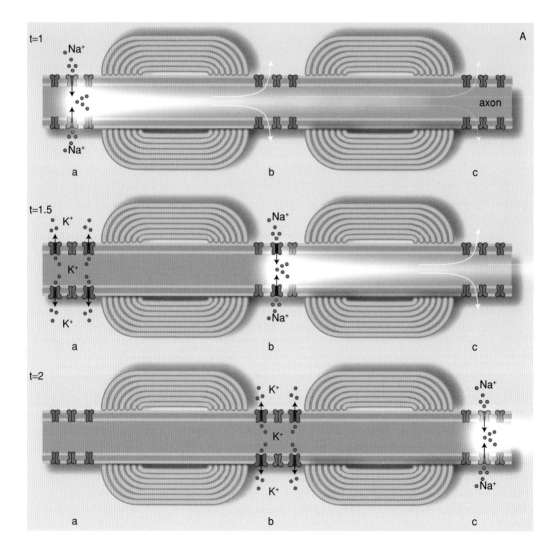

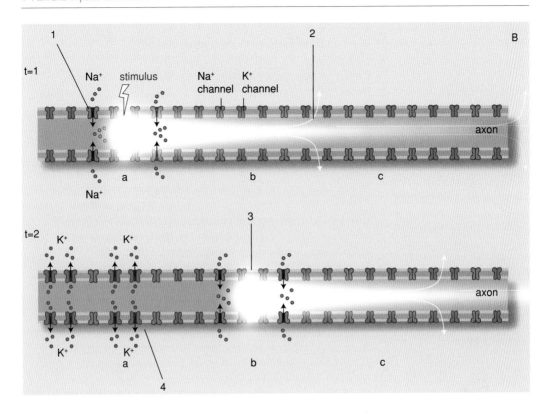

Figure 1.7B
Continuous conduction.

receptors. These postsynaptic receptors consist of ion channels that open once activated, which depolarises the cell membrane, creating an electrical stimulus again, that is propagated along the nerve fibre.

1.2.4   Modulation of the impulse

At the sites where impulses are transferred to other nerves, the impulse stimulus can be enhanced or subdued. This process is called neuromodulation. This can occur both peripherally as well as at connection points in the central nervous system.

One of the most frequent forms of neuromodulation is that affecting the voltage-gated sodium channels involved in the formation and conduction of action potentials. Excitatory neurotransmitters lower the resting potential (hypopolarisation). Consequently, the threshold level can be reached more easily, through which an action potential can occur more quickly. Inhibitory transmitters will only cause an opening of potassium channels, which induces hyperpolarisation of the membrane and an action potential will develop less easily. These mechanisms affect the transmission of impulses. The release of neurotransmitters can also be influenced by presynaptic receptors. Many receptors are involved in these systems, usually selective ion channels (see Box 1.3).

Box 1.3 Modulation of nociceptive stimuli

Various ion channels are involved in the modulation of nociceptive stimuli. They are present, among other places, in the peripheral endings involved in the stimulus perception where they modulate the sensitivity: heat sensitive ion channels (vanilloid receptors, VR1), acid sensitive channels (proton activated receptors) and purine sensitive ion channels (P2X receptors). Besides these, there are also voltage-gated receptors that especially allow passage of sodium or potassium and ligand-gated channels that primarily affect the release of neurotransmitters.

The neurotransmitters are released from the presynaptic nerve ending in large amounts and are able to change the polarity of nerve membranes by opening ion channels. This creates a postsynaptic potential that, depending on the nature, causes either a depolarisation (excitatory postsynaptic potential) or a hyperpolarisation (inhibitory postsynaptic potential). When neurotransmitters open cation channels the nerve is excited (depolarisation). When they open anion channels, inhibition occurs (hyperpolarisation). The most important excitatory neurotransmitter in the nociceptors is glutamate. Substance P plays an important role in peptidergic fibres. Neuropeptides not only have a role in modulating the input to spinal nociceptive neurons and autonomic ganglia, but also cause vasodilation, contraction of smooth muscles, release of histamine from mast cells, chemoattraction of neutrophil granulocytes and proliferation of T lymphocytes and fibroblasts.

Modulation of impulse conduction can also happen through cellular second messengers. An example of this is prostaglandin E_2, which is released during tissue damage. Prostaglandin E_2 increases the sensory transduction via a G protein (protein kinase A). This facilitates the inflow of sodium and the outflow of potassium, changing the electrical charge over the membrane; thus the nerve cell will be stimulated more easily. As a result, a nociceptive stimulus will be propagated more easily. There is, therefore, a local amplification system. On the other hand, afferent fibres exist that have a subduing effect on transduction. For example, activation of μ-receptors (opioids) increases the stimulus threshold that negatively modulates transmission. Pharmacological treatment of pain often intervenes in these modulation systems (Figure 1.8).

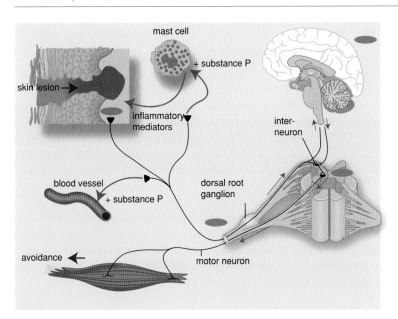

Figure 1.8
Intervention sites for analgesics.

1.3   Perception of pain

Consciousness is a requisite of the perception of pain. Ultimately, the nociceptive stimuli reach the primary sensory cortex, whereby pain is experienced and a physiological response is induced. Pain leads to the release of hormones, such as cortisol and catecholamines, which stimulate the catabolism. Respiration and circulation also increase. Fear and emotion are caused by the transfer of the stimulus to the limbic system.

There are great differences in pain perception between men and women. Women have a lower pain threshold and a lower tolerance for nociceptive stimuli than men. Furthermore, there are great sociocultural differences in the sensation of pain: one patient may experience no pain, while another may cry out from pain, though stimulated by the same stimulus. The emotional state of the patient and environmental factors play an important role in the experience of pain. Fear and excitement have a large influence on the individual pain experience. Fear mobilises the organism to take action in order to avoid or reduce impending damage. As a result, fear causes hypoalgesia. Excitement has the opposite effect.

Aromas have a great impact on mood; this influence is much greater than that of music, which is often used in dental practices in order to influence the sensation of pain. Additionally, the effect of aromas takes place much faster than that of sound or visual stimuli. It has recently been shown that scents, by a change in mood, indeed have a fast and positive influence on the experience of pain.

1.4   Nociception in the orofacial area

The process of transduction, transmission, modulation and perception also occurs in the head and neck area. Tooth pain is caused by stimulation of the polymodal nociceptors in the dental pulp that respond to mechanical and thermal activation. The intensity of the pain is determined by the frequency of the sensory stimulation and by the number of nerve fibres that are excited. Temperature stimulations induce immediate pain responses through the Aδ fibres. When a tooth is stimulated mechanically, fluid moves in the pulpa, which alters the form of the nerve membrane and a stimulus is excited slowly (via C fibres). After application of something cold, the stimulus extinguishes after a while, because vasoconstriction induces lack of oxygen in the nerve. Electrical stimulation induces ion transport, resulting in the stimulation of nerve endings. The same process occurs in osmotic stimulation, for example by sugar and salt. Chemical inflammatory mediators cause the stimulation of nociceptors on the C fibres in the pulpa. Substance P, calcitonin gene-related peptide and neurokinin A have been found in the periodontium and in the pulp of teeth. In painful teeth, the concentration of these inflammatory mediators is increased. They are released from the nerve fibre endings during stimulation and activate the nociceptors. The stimuli are thus propagated by primary Aδ and C fibres, primarily in the trigeminal nerve. At the Gasserian ganglion, they synapse onto secondary fibres that run to the brainstem trigeminal nuclei. From there, they project to the thalamus and the cerebral cortex.

The secondary C fibres end in the most caudal part of the ventrobasal thalamus, run from there to the intralaminar nucleus of the thalamus (forming the activating part of the reticular formation) and project to the cerebral cortex and hypothalamus. The secondary Aδ fibres terminate in the caudal nucleus, where they activate pain tracts to the most caudal part of the ventrobasal thalamus. From there, tertiary tracts run to other parts of the thalamus and somatosensory cortex.

Anatomy of the trigeminal nerve

T.M.G.J. van Eijden and G.E.J. Langenbach

The trigeminal nerve is the fifth cranial nerve (n. V), which plays an important role in the innervation of the head and neck area, together with other cranial and spinal nerves. Knowledge of the nerve's anatomy is very important for the correct application of local anaesthetics.

2.1 Introduction

The trigeminal nerve contains a large number of sensory (afferent) and motor (efferent) neurons. The sensory fibres carry nerve impulses towards the central nervous system, while the motor fibres carry impulses away from the central nervous system. The trigeminal nerve has a wide innervation area (Figure 2.1). The nerve provides the sensitivity of the dentition, the mucosa of the mouth, nose and paranasal sinuses, and the facial skin. The nerve also contains motor fibres that innervate, among

Figure 2.1
Overview of the trigeminal nerve (lateral view).

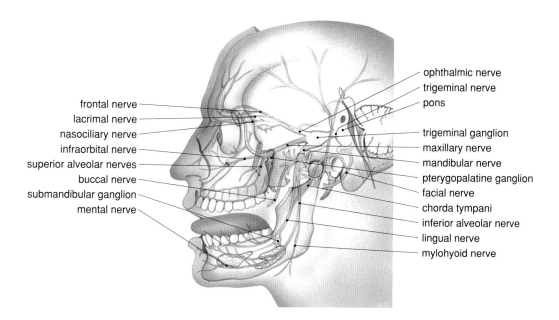

frontal nerve
lacrimal nerve
nasociliary nerve
infraorbital nerve
superior alveolar nerves
buccal nerve
submandibular ganglion
mental nerve

ophthalmic nerve
trigeminal nerve
pons
trigeminal ganglion
maxillary nerve
mandibular nerve
pterygopalatine ganglion
facial nerve
chorda tympani
inferior alveolar nerve
lingual nerve
mylohyoid nerve

others, the masticatory muscles. Although the trigeminal nerve is the most important nerve for the sensory and motor innervation of the oral system, the facial (n. VII), glossopharyngeal (n. IX), vagus (n. X), accessory (n. XI) and hypoglossal (n. XII) nerves are also of significance. The n. VII, n. IX and n. X, for example, take care of the taste sense, the n. IX and n. X provide the general sensation (pain, touch and temperature) to the pharynx, soft palate and the back of the tongue, whilst the n. XII is responsible for the motor innervation of the tongue. Although these latter nerves do play an important role in innervating the oral cavity, they will only be mentioned marginally in this book.

2.2   The central part of the trigeminal nerve

2.2.1   Origin

The trigeminal nerve emerges from the middle of the pons, at the lateral surface of the brainstem. The nerve consists of two parts here: the sensory fibres form a thick root and the motor fibres form the much thinner motor root. These two roots run to the front of the petrous part of the temporal bone where the large sensory trigeminal ganglion (semilunar or Gasserian ganglion) lies in a shallow groove surrounded by dura mater.

   The trigeminal ganglion is formed by the aggregation of cell bodies of sensory neurons. Three main branches of the trigeminal nerve emerge from the ganglion: the ophthalmic nerve (n. V_1), the maxillary nerve (n. V_2) and the mandibular nerve (n. V_3). The motor root joins the mandibular nerve only, once it has exited the skull via the foramen ovale. The sensory areas covered by the three main branches are generally as follows:
- The ophthalmic nerve carries sensory information from the skin of the forehead, the upper eyelids and the nose ridge, and part of the nasal mucosa.
- The maxillary nerve innervates the skin of the middle facial area, the side of the nose and the lower eyelids, the maxillary dentition, part of the nasal mucosa (including the maxillary sinus) and the palate.
- The mandibular nerve innervates the skin of the lower facial area, the mandibular dentition, the mucosa of the lower lip, cheeks and floor of the mouth, part of the tongue and part of the external ear.

Of all the areas that the trigeminal nerve innervates, the oral cavity is the most enriched with sensory neurons. The density of sensory neurons in the mouth is much larger than in any other area, e.g. the facial skin. This density of sensory neurons increases from the back to the frontal area of the mouth.

   Most of the trigeminal ganglion neurons are pseudo-unipolar. This means that each neuron in the ganglion has a peripheral and a central process. The peripheral process (axon) is relatively long and carries the impulses coming from sensory receptors (Box 2.1). The central process (dendrite) is short, and enters the pons and synapses with the sensory trigeminal nucleus situated in the brainstem. The proprioceptive fibres in the trigeminal ganglion are an exception. Their cell bodies are not situated in this ganglion but in the mesencephalic nucleus of the trigeminal nerve. The proprioceptive fibres are found in the motor root of the trigeminal nerve and carry impulses from, among others, muscle spindles of the masticatory muscles.

Box 2.1 Receptors

Sensory nerves are capable of picking up impulses from the external world and the body. The ends of the fibres themselves function as receptors or there are special receptors (e.g. taste receptors, muscle spindles). Each receptor type is the most sensitive to one specific sensation. There are, for example, mechano-receptors (reacting to touch and mild pressure), thermo-receptors (reacting to temperature) and nociceptors (reacting to tissue damage). Nociceptors serve pain sensation. There are also so-called proprioceptors. These are mostly found in muscles (muscle spindles and Golgi tendon organs) and in the joint capsules. They supply information on the position of the jaw and the speed and direction of movement. This form of sensation is called proprioceptive sensibility or proprioception. There are a great number of receptors present in the facial skin and lips, in the mucosa of the oral cavity and tongue, in the teeth and the periodontium, and in the masticatory muscles and temporomandibular joint.

The trigeminal ganglion has somatotopy. This means that the neurons in the ganglion are arranged in the same order as the areas that are innervated by the three main branches of the trigeminal nerve. The cell bodies of the ophthalmic nerve are grouped medially in the ganglion, while those of the mandibular nerve are grouped laterally. In the middle of these two groups the cell bodies of the maxillary nerve can be found.

2.2.2   Trigeminal nuclei

The trigeminal nerve has a sensory and motor nucleus within the brainstem (Figure 2.2). The sensory nucleus lies laterally and most of the sensory neurons of the trigeminal nerve contact (synapse) with the neurons in this nucleus. The nucleus forms a long column that extends from the midbrain to the spinal cord. It consists of (from cranial to caudal) the mesencephalic, the principal and the spinal trigeminal nuclei.

Proprioceptive information from, for example, the masticatory muscles is managed in the mesencephalic nucleus. The principal trigeminal nucleus mainly receives touch and pressure impulses from the entire oral area, whereas the spinal trigeminal nucleus receives information on pain, temperature and pressure from the entire trigeminal area. All information

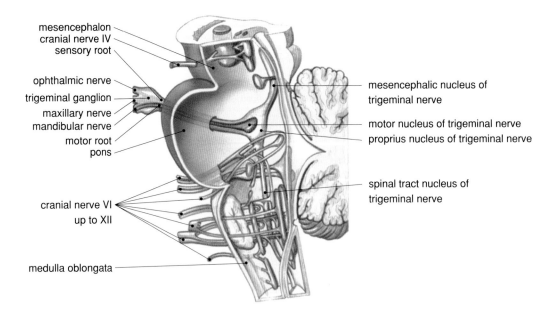

mesencephalon
cranial nerve IV
sensory root

ophthalmic nerve
trigeminal ganglion
maxillary nerve
mandibular nerve
motor root
pons

cranial nerve VI
up to XII

medulla oblongata

mesencephalic nucleus of
trigeminal nerve

motor nucleus of trigeminal nerve
proprius nucleus of trigeminal nerve

spinal tract nucleus of
trigeminal nerve

Figure 2.2

The motor and sensory nuclei of the third to twelfth cranial nerve in the brainstem (lateral view). The sensory nuclei are shown in blue, the motor nuclei in red.

received via the sensory trigeminal nuclei is managed and integrated in, among others, the thalamus via ascending paths. After this the information is brought to various areas of the cerebral cortex, where perception occurs.

The motor neurons of the trigeminal nerve are grouped in a motor nucleus that lies medially to the sensory nucleus in the centre of the pons. The axons of these motor neurons run to (among others) the masticatory muscles. As previously described, these axons pass the trigeminal ganglion as an independent bundle (motor root), without synapsing within it. Similar to the motor neurons in the spinal column, the motor neurons in the motor trigeminal nucleus are directly stimulated via the corticobulbar tract, originating from the contralateral cerebral cortex. Within the motor nucleus there is a large amount of somatotopy, i.e. the motor neurons that innervate the different muscles are grouped together. Via fibres coming from the sensory mesencephalic nucleus, the motor trigeminal nucleus receives proprioceptive information from the masticatory muscles, temporomandibular joint and periodontium.

2.3   The peripheral part of the trigeminal nerve

2.3.1   Ophthalmic nerve

The ophthalmic nerve (n. V$_1$) enters the orbit (Figure 2.3). This nerve carries only sensory fibres and, just before leaving the cranial cavity through the superior orbital fissure, it branches off into three: the nasociliary, frontal and lacrimal nerves. These nerves run in the roof of the orbit and are involved in the sensory innervation of a large number of structures, such as the mucosa of the nasal cavity and the sphenoid and

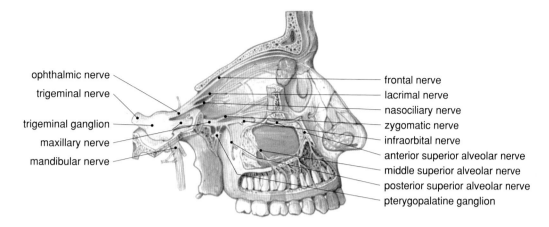

ophthalmic nerve
trigeminal nerve

trigeminal ganglion
maxillary nerve
mandibular nerve

frontal nerve
lacrimal nerve
nasociliary nerve
zygomatic nerve
infraorbital nerve
anterior superior alveolar nerve
middle superior alveolar nerve
posterior superior alveolar nerve
pterygopalatine ganglion

ethmoid sinus, the skin of the nose ridge, the upper eyelid and forehead, and the mucosa that covers the eyeball and inside of the eyelids.

Figure 2.3
The branching of the ophthalmic and maxillary nerves (lateral view).

2.3.2 Maxillary nerve

The maxillary nerve (n. V$_2$), too, is solely sensory. It enters the pterygopalatine fossa (see Section 2.4.1) via the foramen rotundum (Figure 2.3). Through the inferior orbital fissure it reaches the floor of the orbit and proceeds there as the infraorbital nerve, first in the infraorbital sulcus and then in the infraorbital canal. It then reaches the face via the infraorbital foramen.

Within the pterygopalatine fossa the maxillary nerve is connected via a number of branches to the upper side of the parasympathetic pterygopalatine ganglion. Sensory fibres run through these branches which exit on the lower side of the ganglion (Figures 2.4 and 2.5). These sensory fibres form, among others, the following nerves:

• The nasal nerves and nasopalatine nerve that run through the sphenopalatine foramen to the nasal mucosa. The nasal nerves innervate the back part of the nasal mucosa. The nasopalatine nerve, which runs forwards over the nasal septum and reaches the oral cavity through the incisive canal, innervates the frontal part of the palatal mucosa and the palatal gingiva of the maxillary incisors.

• The greater palatine nerve that runs via the greater palatine canal to the mucosa of the hard palate and to the palatal gingiva of the maxillary alveolar process.

• The lesser palatine nerves that run to the mucosa of the soft palate via the lesser palatine canals.

Together with the palatine nerves there are also parasympathetic and orthosympathetic fibres that run from the pterygopalatine ganglion to the salivary glands in the palatal mucosa.

In the pterygopalatine fossa the maxillary nerve also branches into the posterior superior alveolar nerve and the zygomatic nerve (Figure 2.3).

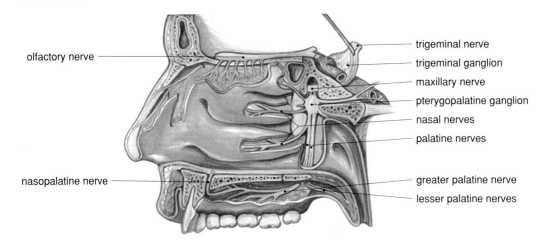

olfactory nerve

trigeminal nerve

trigeminal ganglion

maxillary nerve

pterygopalatine ganglion

nasal nerves

palatine nerves

nasopalatine nerve

greater palatine nerve

lesser palatine nerves

Figure 2.4
The maxillary nerve
(medial view).

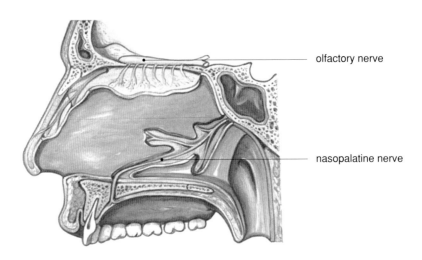

olfactory nerve

nasopalatine nerve

Figure 2.5
The path of the nasopalatine
nerve over the nasal septum.

The posterior superior alveolar nerve exits the pterygopalatine fossa
through the pterygomaxillary fissure and runs over the maxillary
tuberosity. The nerve divides into a large number of little branches,
the posterior superior alveolar rami, which enter the wall of the maxilla
through small openings and innervate the maxillary molars and
corresponding buccal gingiva. The zygomatic nerve arrives in the orbit via
the inferior orbital fissure and branches into the zygomaticotemporal and
zygomaticofacial nerves. These exit the lateral orbital wall through small
canals in the zygomatic bone and innervate the skin above. The zygomatic
nerve also contains postganglionic parasympathetic fibres that come from
the pterygopalatine ganglion and that join the lacrimal nerve (branch
of n. V_1) for the lacrimal gland.

As it runs along the orbital floor the infraorbital nerve branches into two: the middle superior alveolar nerve, for the innervation of the maxillary premolars and the corresponding buccal gingiva, and the anterior superior alveolar nerve, for the maxillary canine and incisors and the corresponding buccal gingiva. These nerves usually run between the mucosa and outer wall of the maxillary sinus. There they divide into a number of small branches, the medial and anterior superior alveolar rami that penetrate into the maxillary alveolar process via small openings. Inside the bone they form together with the posterior superior alveolar rami, right above the apices, an extensive nervous network – the superior alveolar plexus – from which short little branches are sent to the dentition and gingiva.

Once the infraorbital nerve reaches the face via the infraorbital foramen, it splits into a large number of branches for the sensory innervation of the skin of the lower eyelid (palpebral rami), the infraorbital region, the side of the nose (nasal rami) and the skin and mucosa of the upper lip (labial rami).

2.3.3 Mandibular nerve

The mandibular nerve (n. V_3) contains both sensory and motor fibres. This nerve exits the skull through the foramen ovale and ends in the infratemporal fossa (see Section 2.4.2; Figure 2.6). The mandibular nerve runs between the lateral pterygoid muscle and the tensor veli palatini muscle. The nerve sends a motor branch to the latter muscle.

The mandibular nerve splits into two main branches, the anterior and posterior trunks. From the anterior trunk a sensory nerve emerges, the buccal nerve, and a number of motor nerves, i.e. the pterygoid nerves, the deep temporal nerves and the masseteric nerve. Three branches emerge from the posterior trunk: the auriculotemporal nerve (sensory), the inferior alveolar nerve (mixed sensory and motor) and the lingual nerve (sensory).

Figure 2.6

The mandibular nerve (lateral view).

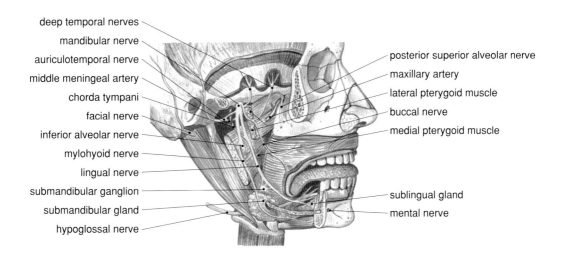

The buccal nerve runs along the medial surface of the upper head of the lateral pterygoid muscle and moves laterally between the two heads of the muscle. The nerve innervates the skin and mucosa of the cheek and the buccal gingiva of the mandibular alveolar process at the level of the molars and premolars.

The pterygoid nerves are short motor branches for the medial and lateral pterygoid muscles. The masseteric nerve runs laterally along the top of the upper head of the lateral pterygoid muscle and reaches the deep surface of the masseter muscle via the mandibular notch. The deep temporal nerves also run high along the lateral pterygoid muscle and penetrate the medial side of the temporal muscle.

The auriculotemporal nerve arises as two roots encircling the middle meningeal artery. The nerve first runs laterally behind the mandibular neck and then bends upwards in front of the ear. It is involved in the sensory innervation of the temporomandibular joint and the skin of the temporal and auricle region. The nerve also contains postganglionic parasympathetic fibres for the parotid gland from the otic ganglion. This parasympathetic ganglion lies between the mandibular nerve and the tensor veli palatini.

At its origin, the inferior alveolar nerve contains motor and sensory fibres. It runs deep to the lateral pterygoid muscle. Emerging from beneath this muscle it directs to the mandibular foramen. Just before it enters the mandibular canal it gives off its motor mylohyoid branch for the mylohyoid muscle and for the anterior belly of the digastric muscle. Inside the mandibular canal the inferior alveolar nerve contains only sensory fibres. Here, under the apices, a network is formed, the inferior alveolar plexus, from which little branches are sent to the dentition and gingiva (Figure 2.7). Anteriorly, the inferior alveolar nerve gives off the mental nerve. This emerges from the mental foramen and innervates the skin of the chin, the skin and mucosa of the lower lip and the buccal

Figure 2.7

The innervation of the dentition by the superior alveolar nerves and the inferior alveolar nerve.

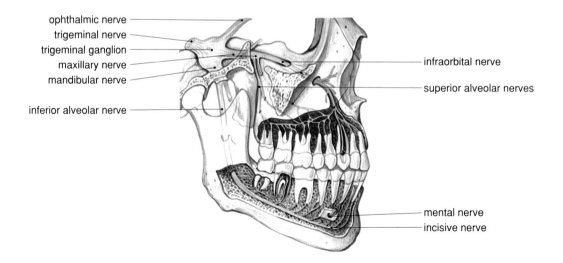

ophthalmic nerve
trigeminal nerve
trigeminal ganglion
maxillary nerve
mandibular nerve

inferior alveolar nerve

infraorbital nerve

superior alveolar nerves

mental nerve
incisive nerve

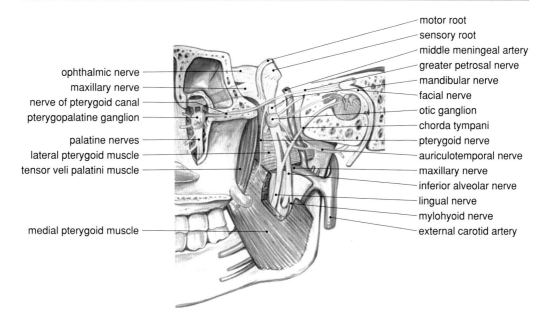

ophthalmic nerve
maxillary nerve
nerve of pterygoid canal
pterygopalatine ganglion
palatine nerves
lateral pterygoid muscle
tensor veli palatini muscle
medial pterygoid muscle

motor root
sensory root
middle meningeal artery
greater petrosal nerve
mandibular nerve
facial nerve
otic ganglion
chorda tympani
pterygoid nerve
auriculotemporal nerve
maxillary nerve
inferior alveolar nerve
lingual nerve
mylohyoid nerve
external carotid artery

Figure 2.8
The mandibular nerve (medial view).

gingiva of the inferior alveolar process at the level of the canine and incisors. The last stretch of the inferior alveolar nerve inside the mandibular canal that runs in the direction of the symphysis is usually named as a separate nerve, the incisive nerve.

The lingual nerve is joined, directly after its separation of n. V_3, by the chorda tympani (Figure 2.8). This is a branch of the facial nerve with preganglionic parasympathetic fibres from the brainstem and sensory nerves for the taste of the anterior two-thirds of the tongue (Box 2.2). The lingual nerve runs deep to the lateral pterygoid muscle and forwards over the lateral surface of the medial pterygoid muscle. At the level of the apices of the third mandibular molar it lies immediately beneath the mucosa

---

Box 2.2 Innervation of the tongue

Various nerves are involved in the sensory and motor innervation of the tongue. The general sensitivity (pain, touch, temperature) of the anterior two-thirds of the tongue is supplied by the lingual nerve (branch of the n. V_3). The specific sensitivity (taste) of the anterior two-thirds is supplied by the chorda tympani (branch of the n. VII). Because the chorda tympani joins the lingual nerve high up in the infratemporal fossa, these taste fibres reach the tongue together with the lingual nerve. The sensitivity, general and specific, of the posterior third of the tongue is supplied by the glossopharyngeal nerve (n. IX). The motor innervation of the tongue takes place through the hypoglossal nerve (n. XII).

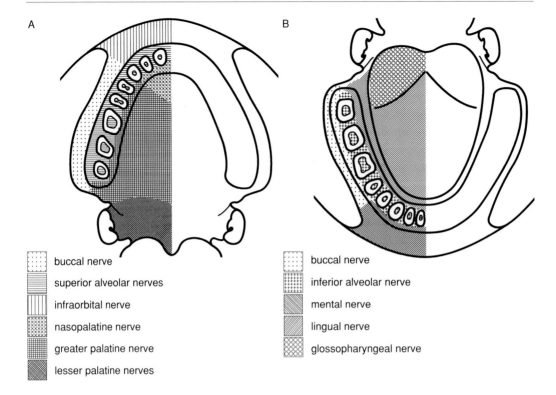

A

buccal nerve

superior alveolar nerves

infraorbital nerve

nasopalatine nerve

greater palatine nerve

lesser palatine nerves

B

buccal nerve

inferior alveolar nerve

mental nerve

lingual nerve

glossopharyngeal nerve

Figure 2.9 A and B

The sensory innervation of the oral cavity. **A** The palate, the superior alveolar process, the cheek and the upper lip. **B** The tongue, the inferior alveolar process, the cheek and the lower lip.

against the inner side of the mandible. It continues superiorly to the mylohyoid muscle, passing under the submandibular duct, and then ascends in the tongue. The section of the lingual nerve that comes from n. V_3 supplies the general sensitivity (pain, touch, temperature) of the anterior two-thirds of the tongue, the mucosa of the floor of the mouth and the lingual gingiva of the inferior alveolar process. The submandibular parasympathetic ganglion is closely related to the lingual nerve. This ganglion is connected by a number of small branches to the underside of the nerve. Preganglionic parasympathetic fibres from the chorda tympani reach the ganglion via these branches. The postganglionic parasympathetic fibres run to the submandibular and sublingual glands.

A schematic summary of the sensory innervation of the oral cavity with the areas supplied by the various branches of the maxillary and mandibular nerves is given in Figure 2.9.

2.4   Deep areas

The pterygopalatine fossa and the infratemporal fossa (including the pterygomandibular space) are deep areas in the head that are of great significance for block anaesthesia of (branches of) the maxillary and mandibular nerves respectively.

2.4.1   Pterygopalatine fossa

The pterygopalatine fossa is a small pyramid-shaped space that lies medially to the infratemporal fossa. The tip of the pyramid is directed downwards. The fossa is found behind the orbit and the maxillary tuberosity and also lateral to the posterior part of the nasal cavity. The posterior wall is formed by the pterygoid process of the sphenoid bone, the medial wall by the perpendicular plate of the palatine bone and the anterior wall by the maxillary tuberosity.

The pterygopalatine fossa has a large number of openings and forms an important junction for blood vessels and nerves. In the top of the fossa the cranial cavity can be accessed posteriorly via the foramen rotundum, and it is connected anteriorly via the medial part of the inferior orbital fissure to the orbit. Laterally the infratemporal fossa can be reached via the triangular, narrow pterygomaxillary fissure. Medially the sphenopalatine foramen forms the connection with the nasal cavity. The downwards directed tip of the fossa runs narrowly to the greater palatine canal, thus reaching the palate.

The maxillary artery reaches the pterygopalatine fossa through the pterygomaxillary fissure. Within the fossa the artery gives off various branches:
- The posterior superior alveolar artery and the infraorbital artery that run alongside the veins and nerves of the same name.
- The descending palatine artery that runs downwards through the greater palatine canal and splits into the greater palatine artery and the lesser palatine arteries. The greater palatine artery runs forwards over the hard palate, whereas the lesser palatine arteries serve the soft palate (Figure 2.10).
- The sphenopalatine artery that runs through the sphenopalatine foramen to the mucosa of the nasal cavity.

Veins, which drain regions supplied by these arteries, connect with the pterygoid plexus.

As mentioned previously, the maxillary nerve enters the pterygopalatine fossa via the foramen rotundum. The nerve runs forwards along the top side of the fossa and enters the orbit via the inferior orbital fissure. From this point the nerve is called the infraorbital nerve. In the fossa, the maxillary nerve gives off the posterior superior alveolar nerve that leaves the fossa through the pterygomaxillary fissure and uses the surface of the maxillary tuberosity to reach the maxillary molars. Immediately beneath the maxillary nerve lies the pterygopalatine ganglion, which serves, among others, the parasympathetic innervation of the lacrimal gland, salivary glands of the palate, and mucous glands in the nasal cavity, using the various branches of the maxillary nerve. The orthosympathetic innervation of these structures originates from the superior cervical ganglion which branches into a network around the arteries of the head region. The maxillary nerve also branches off downwards in the greater and lesser palatine nerves, which contain sensory fibres for the hard and soft palate respectively; they leave the pterygopalatine fossa via the greater

Figure 2.10
The palate from below.

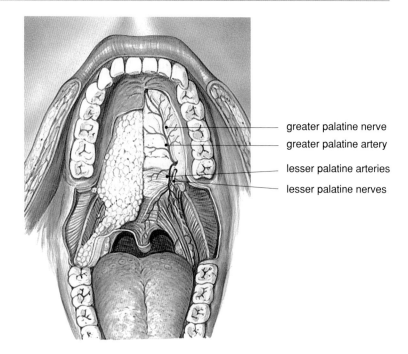

greater palatine nerve
greater palatine artery
lesser palatine arteries
lesser palatine nerves

palatine foramen and the lesser palatine foramina. Medially the maxillary nerve branches off into the nasopalatine nerve, for the innervation of the nasal cavity via the sphenopalatine foramen. This nerve eventually also reaches the anterior part of the palate via the nasal septum and the incisive canal.

2.4.2   Infratemporal fossa and pterygomandibular space

The infratemporal fossa is an area on the inner side of the zygomatic arch and the mandibular ramus. The other bony boundaries of the fossa are the greater wing of the sphenoid bone on the upper side, the maxillary tuberosity on the anterior side and the lateral plate of the pterygoid process (sphenoid bone) on the medial side. The pharynx wall provides a soft tissue boundary, medially and ventrally.

On the posterior side, the infratemporal fossa changes, without a clear border, into the parapharyngeal and retropharyngeal space. Medially the fossa provides access to the pterygopalatine fossa via the pterygomaxillary fissure. The fossa is connected via the foramen ovale and the foramen spinosum to the cranial cavity, and via the lateral part of the inferior orbital fissure it is connected to the orbit.

The lateral pterygoid muscle and the medial pterygoid muscle are situated within this fossa (Figure 2.11). Besides these muscles the infratemporal fossa is filled to a large extent by a fat body that is an extenuation of the buccal fat pad (of Bichat). Blood vessels and nerves are embedded within this fat, i.e. the maxillary artery, the pterygoid venous plexus, the mandibular nerve and all of their branches.

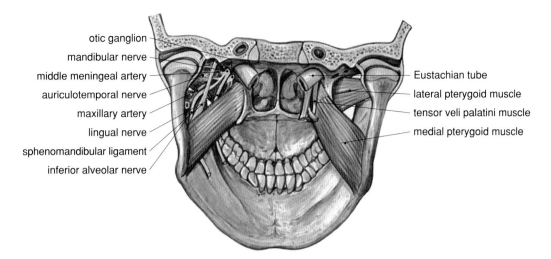

otic ganglion
mandibular nerve
middle meningeal artery
auriculotemporal nerve
maxillary artery
lingual nerve
sphenomandibular ligament
inferior alveolar nerve

Eustachian tube
lateral pterygoid muscle
tensor veli palatini muscle
medial pterygoid muscle

The lateral and medial pterygoid muscles, together with the mandibular ramus, border a separate space within the infratemporal fossa, the so-called pterygomandibular space. In a frontal cross section, the pterygomandibular space is triangular in shape, enclosed medially by the medial pterygoid muscle, cranially by the lateral pterygoid muscle and laterally by the mandibular ramus. The space is bordered ventrally by the pharynx wall and dorsally by the deep section of the parotid gland (Figure 2.12). The space merges into the submandibular space ventro-caudally and more medially and caudo-cranially it merges into the parapharyngeal and retropharyngeal spaces, which eventually convert into the mediastinum.

The most important artery in the infratemporal fossa is the maxillary artery (Figure 2.13). This artery supplies blood to the nasal cavity, the palate, the maxilla and mandible and the masticatory muscles. The artery

Figure 2.11
The infratemporal fossa viewed from behind.

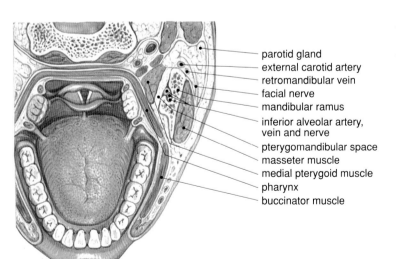

parotid gland
external carotid artery
retromandibular vein
facial nerve
mandibular ramus
inferior alveolar artery, vein and nerve
pterygomandibular space
masseter muscle
medial pterygoid muscle
pharynx
buccinator muscle

Figure 2.12
Horizontal cross section of the oral cavity and of the pterygomandibular space.

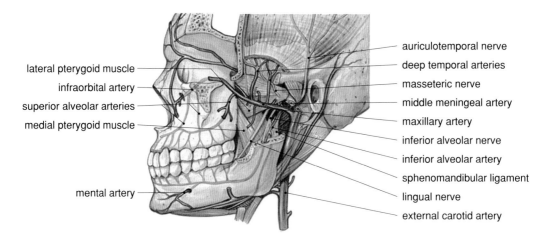

lateral pterygoid muscle
infraorbital artery
superior alveolar arteries
medial pterygoid muscle

mental artery

auriculotemporal nerve
deep temporal arteries
masseteric nerve
middle meningeal artery
maxillary artery
inferior alveolar nerve
inferior alveolar artery
sphenomandibular ligament
lingual nerve
external carotid artery

Figure 2.13

The maxillary artery
(lateral view).

enters the fossa between the mandibular neck and the sphenomandibular ligament. It subsequently runs to the lower margin of the lateral pterygoid muscle and continues medially or laterally from this muscle to the pterygopalatine fossa. Besides giving off a large number of branches to muscles (masseteric artery, deep temporal arteries, pterygoid arteries), the maxillary artery also branches off, among others, the middle meningeal artery, which reaches the cranial cavity via the foramen spinosum, and the inferior alveolar artery. The latter nerve enters, together with the inferior alveolar vein and nerve, the mandibular canal via the mandibular foramen and supplies blood to the lower jaw. The mental artery, which branches off from the inferior alveolar artery at the end of the mandibular canal, exits with the mental vein and nerve through the mental foramen and supplies blood to the chin and lower lip. Within the infratemporal fossa, the veins continue to follow the path of the arteries. These veins lead into the extensive pterygoid venous plexus, which lies against the lateral pterygoid muscle. The pterygoid plexus connects posteriorly, via the short maxillary vein, with the retromandibular vein, and anteriorly with the facial vein.

The mandibular nerve reaches the infratemporal fossa via the foramen ovale. The parasympathetic otic ganglion, which innervates, among others, the parotid gland and the salivary glands in the cheek, lies directly under the foramen ovale, on the medial side of the nerve. This nerve initially runs between the medial side of the lateral pterygoid muscle and the medial pterygoid muscle and gives off motor branches here for the innervation of the lateral and medial pterygoid muscles (pterygoid nerves), the temporalis muscle (deep temporal nerves), the masseter muscle (masseteric nerve), and the tensor tympani and tensor veli palatini muscles. Sensory branches are the buccal, lingual, inferior alveolar and auriculotemporal nerves. The buccal nerve runs laterally between the two heads of the lateral pterygoid muscle and then continues to the cheek. This nerve also contains parasympathetic fibres for the innervation of the salivary glands. The auriculotemporal nerve initially consists of two roots, which pass around the medial meningeal artery. The auriculotemporal nerve runs in a dorsolateral direction to the mandibular neck, continues behind it and innervates, among others, the temporomandibular joint, the skin behind this joint and the skin in front of the ear. This nerve also contains parasympathetic fibres for the parotid gland, which originate from the otic ganglion. The two largest branches of the mandibular nerve are the inferior alveolar nerve and the lingual nerve. These two nerves first run medially from the lateral pterygoid muscle. On the medial side of this muscle, the chorda tympani also joins the lingual nerve. The two nerves enter the pterygomandibular space at the lower margin of the lateral pterygoid muscle.

Pharmacology of local anaesthetics

A.L. Frankhuijzen

Local anaesthetics are the most commonly used pharmaceuticals in dentistry. They interfere reversibly with the generation of the action potential and with cellular impulse conduction by blockading the sodium channels in the nerve cell. This results in a local insensibility to pain stimuli.

3.1 Classification

Local anaesthetics share several common characteristics in their molecular structure (Figure 3.1). A lipophilic group can be identified which determines lipid solubility. Another part contains a hydrophilic group that determines the degree of water solubility. Usually the lipophilic part of the molecule is an aromatic structure that contains a benzene ring. The hydrophilic part contains a secondary or a tertiary amine. Both parts, present at the opposite ends of the molecule, are connected by an intermediate section. This intermediate section consists of an ester or an amide group and a relatively short chain of four to five carbon atoms (Box 3.1).

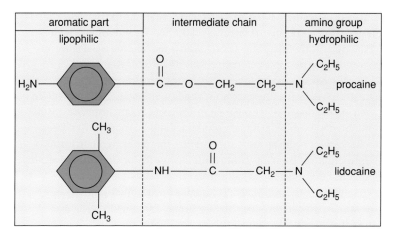

Figure 3.1

Molecular structure of an ester-linked (procaine) and amide-linked local anaesthetic (lidocaine). (Modified from Borchard (1985) *Aktuelle Aspekte der Zahnärzlichen Lokalanasthesie*. Hoechst AG.)

Box 3.1

In general, carbon groups can be added to each of the three parts of the molecule (up to a certain maximum). These alterations in molecular structure result in local anaesthetics with strongly different pharmacokinetic properties, since this changes the degree of protein binding, the lipid solubility and the way the local anaesthetic is eliminated. This may result in large differences in onset time, duration of action and effectiveness of local anaesthesia (Table B3.1).

Table B3.1	An overview of regularly used local anaesthetics with average values of onset time, duration of action and effectiveness relative to prilocaine.		
	Onset of action after	*Duration of action*	*Effectiveness*
Articaine	5 min	1–3 hours	3
Bupivacaine	8 min	3–7 hours	16
Lidocaine	5 min	$\frac{1}{2}$–2 hours	4
Mepivacaine	3 min	2–2$\frac{1}{2}$ hours	2
Prilocaine	2 min	$\frac{1}{2}$–1 hour	1

The data presented have only meaning for comparison purposes. In dental practice, these factors strongly depend on the location and method of administration.

In other words, local anaesthetics can be classified according to their molecular structure into two classes: the (amino-) esters and the (amino-) amides. Both groups differ in the way in which they are metabolised.

In ester anaesthetics, the aromatic part containing the benzene ring is derived from para amino benzoic acid (PABA). The intermediate chain, characteristic for this group, contains an ester-binding (see Figure 3.1). A well-known example of an ester-anaesthetic is procaine.

Amide-anaesthetics have been developed more recently and are characterised by the presence of an amide-binding in the intermediate chain, as in lidocaine (see Figure 3.1). The amides can further be divided into three subgroups: xylidines, toluidines and thiophenes. Xylidines are tertiary amines with an aromatic part that contains two methyl groups. Representatives from this group are lidocaine (Xylocaine®), mepivacaine (Scandicaine®) and bupivacaine (Marcaine®) (Box 3.2).

In toluidines, the benzene ring contains a single methyl group and the amine part contains a secondary amine. A frequently used local anaesthetic from this group is prilocaine (Citanest®).

> **Box 3.2**
>
> The tertiary amine part of mepivacaine contains a piperidine ring with a methyl group attached, instead of two methyl groups. Bupivacaine also contains a piperidine ring but with a butyl group attached. This butyl group is responsible for the stronger local anaesthetic effect of bupivacaine and the very long duration of action of this local anaesthetic (Table B3.1).

Thiophenes, such as articaine (Ultracain®; Septanest®), have a slightly different molecular structure. They contain a sulphur ring in the aromatic part of the molecule. This is probably the reason why this local anaesthetic has a better penetration into the mucosa and the jaw bone as well.

3.2 Pharmacodynamics

Local anaesthetics differ considerably in onset time, duration of action and strength of the analgesic effect. The strength of the local anaesthetic effect is directly related to the lipid solubility of the local anaesthetic.

Of the series bupivacaine–articaine–lidocaine–prilocaine–mepivacaine, the first anaesthetic is the most lipid soluble and the last one the least. The same order applies to the strength of the analgesic effect of these compounds (Box 3.3). The differences in analgesic strength of the compounds, however, seem smaller than theoretically expected (see table in Box 3.1). Probably, pharmacokinetic aspects are also important for the strength of the analgesic effect. An overview of factors that can affect the intrinsic activity of local anaesthetics is presented in Table 3.1.

Table 3.1	Some factors that affect the intrinsic properties of local anaesthetics.
Factor	*Mechanism*
Pregnancy	Progesterone can potentiate the nerve blocking effect of the local anaesthetic.
pH alteration	Inflammation and uraemia lower the tissue pH. This reduces the percentage of the neutral base form. A pH alteration can also affect the binding to plasma and tissue proteins, and seems relevant for the rapid appearance of tolerance during a repeat injection.
Vasodilatation	Intrinsic vasodilatation causes rapid elimination from the area of injection. For example, bupivacaine is a vasodilator.
Vasoconstriction	A vasoconstrictor masks the inherent vasodilatory properties of the local anaesthetic and causes an increased effect that also lasts longer.

Box 3.3

The potency of a local anaesthetic is expressed by the parameter C_m, defined as the minimum concentration of local anaesthetic required to reduce the amplitude of the action potential by 50% within 5 minutes in a solution with pH 7.2–7.4 and a stimulus frequency of 30 Hz. Of course, this parameter can only be determined with in vitro experiments.

3.3   Pharmacokinetics

3.3.1   Physical–chemical characteristics

Local anaesthetics are weak bases, unstable and poorly water soluble. With a single exception, they are tertiary amines. Therefore hydrochloric acid (HCl) is added to the local anaesthetic, which converts the tertiary amine, expressed below as R_3N, into a chloride salt:

$$R_3N + HCl \rightarrow R_3NH^+ + Cl^-$$

This increases the stability and water solubility of a local anaesthetic:

$$R_3NH^+ + H_2O \overset{K_a}{\leftrightarrow} R_3N + H_3O^+$$

In which R_3NH^+ represents the water-soluble, ionised, quaternary cation form of the local anaesthetic, which is responsible for the analgesic effect. This 'active' form is in equilibrium with the 'inactive' form, the uncharged tertiary base R_3N (Boxes 3.4 and 3.5). The equilibrium constant K_a of most local anaesthetics is between 7 and 8.

3.3.2   Diffusion

From the site of administration, a local anaesthetic must cross several barriers to reach the actual site of action. For this, the uncharged base form of the local anaesthetic is necessary (R_3N). This form is lipophilic (fat soluble), enabling it to pass through the cell membrane of neurons. The fat solubility of a local anaesthetic is primarily determined by the charge of the molecule and – to a lesser extent – by the length of the molecule skeleton: the longer the chain, the greater the fat solubility.

   Once the uncharged lipophilic form is inside the cell, a new equilibrium with the water-soluble charged form will be established. The intracellular pH is lower than outside, so the equilibrium will shift towards R_3NH^+, the active cationic form of the anaesthetic. Consequently, the proportion between both forms (R_3N and R_3NH^+) plays an essential role in the function of local anaesthetics.

Box 3.4

The relative proportion of the base (R_3N) and cationic form (R_3NH^+) depend on the pK_a (the dissociation constant of the local anaesthetic), the pH of the solution and the pH at the site of injection, as defined by the Henderson-Hasselbalch equation:

$$\log (C_i/C_o) = pK_a - pH$$

In this equation, C_i represents the concentration local anaesthetic in the active, ionised cationic form (R_3NH^+) and C_o the concentration of the inactive, unionised base form (R_3N). When the pH at the site of injection has the same value as the pK_a, 50% of the local anaesthetic will be present in the unionised form. With a low pH at the injection site, e.g. an injection into inflamed tissue, the percentage of the unionised form will be less than half. Under this condition, less local anaesthetic will be available for diffusion through the lipid membrane to the inside of the nerve cell. This means that the dose administered will analgesically be less effective than assumed based on the dose injected.

The pK_as of some regularly used local anaesthetics are presented in Table 3.2.

Box 3.5

Local anaesthetics are less effective in inflamed areas. Only the unionised, lipophilic form of a local anaesthetic is able to cross the cell membrane. The addition of HCl results in a solution of local anaesthetic with a pH of 4–6. Due to the presence of these protons, the equilibrium reaction shifts to the right and the ionised form of the local anaesthetic will dominate. After the administration, the buffering capacity of the tissues returns the pH to the normal value of 7.4. At this pH, the equilibrium returns to the left, which increases the concentration of unionised local anaesthetic. The acid environment that occurs in inflamed tissues results in a low tissue pH. Therefore, the local anaesthetic will present predominantly in the ionised form, which is not able to cross the membrane and consequently local anaesthetics are less effective in inflamed tissues. In addition, the hyperaemia present in inflamed tissues will carry away the local anaesthetic at an increased rate.

A similar mechanism operates during the administration of a repeat injection of an additional amount of local anaesthetic. When the dentist notices that the anaesthesia is not sufficient, the injection of an additional (large) amount of local anaesthetic will create an acid environment, since the injection fluid itself has a pH of 4–6.

Table 3.2	A local anaesthetic with a different pK$_a$ or a change in pH affects the percentage of anaesthetic present in the unionised, inactive base form.			
	pK$_a$	pH = 7.0	pH = 7.4	pH = 7.8
Articaine	7.8	13	29	50
Bupivacaine	8.1	7	17	33
Lidocaine	7.7	17	33	55

It generally applies that the closer the pK$_a$ value of an anaesthetic to the pH of the injection site, the higher the concentration (C$_0$) of the uncharged base form (R$_3$N) of the molecule which is necessary for the diffusion and penetration of the nerve membrane. Choosing a local anaesthetic with a low pK$_a$ or increasing the pH of the local anaesthetic solution will increase the percentage of the lipid-soluble uncharged form of the molecule. This is presented in Table 3.2, which lists the percentages of uncharged base form of three local anaesthetics at different pHs.

However, for the spread from the administration site to the site of action, a local anaesthetic must have a certain degree of water solubility. For this diffusion in the interstitial fluid between the cells, the water-soluble ionised form (R$_3$NH$^+$) is important.

Therefore, both forms of the local anaesthetic, the unionised lipophilic base form (R$_3$N) and the hydrophilic ionised form (R$_3$NH$^+$), must be present in sufficient amounts. This is embedded in their characteristics of being a weak base, where both forms of the local anaesthetic are in equilibrium.

3.3.3   Mode of action of local anaesthetics

Local anaesthetics block the development of an action potential and conduction in the cell membrane. They achieve this by inhibiting the voltage-dependent increase in sodium conductivity over the cell membrane.

It is generally assumed that the most frequently used local anaesthetics act by a combination of membrane expansion and blockade of the sodium channels on the inside of the neuron. The uncharged, lipophilic form of the anaesthetic (R$_3$N) penetrates the lipid part of the membrane, producing a structural change of the lipid bilayer which disturbs the conduction in the membrane of the neuron. This so-called membrane expansion is responsible for approximately 10% of the total activity of most local anaesthetics.

The remaining 90% of the activity depends on an interaction between the charged cationic form of the molecule (R$_3$NH$^+$) and the phospholipid phosphatidyl-L-serine in the neuronal membrane. This interaction causes a disturbance of the calcium binding, with the closure of the sodium channel as a result. The strength of the effect of local anaesthetics on sodium channels is dependent on the frequency of the action potential. On the one hand, when the sodium channel is open it is more accessible for the local anaesthetic. On the other hand, local anaesthetics have a higher affinity with open sodium channels.

The total process is called conduction blockade or membrane stabilisation and consists of a decrease in sodium conduction and a reduction in the rate of depolarisation. In addition, the threshold potential level will no longer be reached, so an action potential cannot occur anymore. However, the resting potential, the threshold potential and the repolarisation of the cell membrane will not or hardly be affected.

3.3.4 Protein binding

Local anaesthetics bind reversibly to both plasma and tissue proteins. They bind primarily to globulins, erythrocytes and less to plasma albumin. Bupivacaine and articaine are strongly bound to plasma proteins (>90%); mepivacaine, lidocaine and prilocaine are less strongly bound (80, 60 and 55%, respectively).

The degree of protein binding is a determining factor for the duration time of a local anaesthetic. In general, the higher the degree of binding to plasma proteins, the longer the local anaesthetic will be active. The plasma protein bound fraction of the local anaesthetic functions as a depot, from which the free local anaesthetic can be released. Remarkably, prilocaine, with a relatively low degree of binding to plasma proteins, binds strongly to tissue proteins, so potentially a toxic concentration will be reached less easily (owing to a larger distribution volume).

3.3.5 Onset time and duration of action

The onset time and the duration of action of local anaesthetics can vary considerably (Box 3.6). In general, the lower the pK_a of a local anaesthetic (or the higher the pH at the injection site), the shorter the onset time. This is a direct result of the increase in the concentration of the unionised, lipophilic form of the local anaesthetic (see Table 3.2). With identical pK_as the degree of lipid solubility is the determining factor: the higher the lipid solubility, the shorter the onset time.

In addition to the characteristics mentioned above, the total dose (in milligrammes) directly determines the onset time (at clinically used dosages). The volume determines the spread. Finally, the concentration determines the strength of the local anaesthetic effect.

The determining factor for the duration of the local analgesic effect is diffusion from the site of administration, followed by redistribution throughout the tissues. In this, the blood flow is the most important factor. Therefore both the total dose and the lipid solubility as well as the presence of a vasoconstrictor affect the duration time. Doubling the dose does not increase the duration time by a factor of two, but only by one

---

Box 3.6

The diameter and myelination varies among the different type of
nerve fibres, which affects the order in which they are being blocked.
After administration of a local anaesthetic around a peripheral nerve,
first stimulus conduction is inhibited in the least myelinated fibres,
especially in the preganglionic autonomic B fibres. This inhibits the
vasoconstrictive activity of these nerve fibres, resulting in vasodilatation
and an increased skin temperature. Next, inhibition of pain and
temperature perception will follow, due to blockade of the Aδ and
C fibres.

   The function of the Aγ and Aβ fibres – responsible for proprioception
and touch and pressure perception – is switched off last of all or, in some
cases, remains intact. The latter sometimes induces a very unpleasant
sensation in patients. During dental treatment, the patient does not
feel pain but will experience the touch of the dentist. In most cases,
explanation and information will relieve complaints that may arise
from this strange phenomenon. Finally and eventually, the motor
Aα fibres are blocked.

---

half-life time. The addition of a vasoconstrictor to the local anaesthetic is
the most important factor in increasing the duration time of short- and
intermediate-acting local anaesthetics, such as lidocaine and articaine.

3.3.6 Local elimination

Finally, local anaesthetic is removed from the site of administration by
the blood, where the degree of vascularisation of the tissue determines
the amount and velocity. Inherent characteristics of the local anaesthetic
(such as vasodilatation) and the total injected dose are additional
determining factors.

   If a local anaesthetic is administered without a vasoconstrictor, it will
disappear from the site of administration in three phases. The initial rapid
α phase represents redistribution by the general circulation from the site
of administration to vessel-rich tissues; the slower β phase represents
redistribution to tissues with less blood supply, while the slowest γ phase
represents the metabolism and excretion of the local anaesthetic. In
general, these three phases are shorter for high lipophilic and low protein
bound local anaesthetics. Table 3.3 shows the half-lives of the three phases
for some frequently used local anaesthetics. These characteristics also
depend on the physical condition of the patient. For example, a patient
with heart failure has a slower α and β phase and – partly therefore – a
slower metabolisation and excretion (γ phase).

   From Table 3.3 it is clear that prilocaine has the fastest redistribution
phases (α and β phases) as well as the highest clearance and metabolism in

Table 3.3	Half-life values of the three phases of plasma elimination of local anaesthetics in healthy individuals.		
	α phase (sec)	β phase (min)	γ phase (hour)
Articaine	30	102	1.3
Bupivacaine	160	200	3.5
Lidocaine	60	96	1.5
Mepivacaine	40	114	2.0
Prilocaine	29	93	1.2

the lungs and kidneys (γ phase). Furthermore, prilocaine has the lowest inherent vasodilator activity and the lowest binding to plasma proteins, the latter resulting in a large distribution volume. The result of all these factors is that prilocaine is 60% less toxic than all other local anaesthetics. However, prilocaine has one disadvantage: it is a toluidine derivative, and during degradation of toluidines the metabolite orthotoluidine is generated. This orthotoluidine can oxidise the Fe^{2+} in haemoglobin to Fe^{3+}, which reduces the oxygen transport capacity, and methaemoglobinaemia develops (see Box 11.1).

3.3.7   Systemic elimination

The aromatic part of the ester-type local anaesthetics is derived from para amino benzoic acid (PABA). Ester anaesthetics are metabolised in plasma by the enzyme pseudo cholinesterase, which generates PABA analogues and amino alcohol. The PABA analogues are excreted in the urine mainly unaltered; the amino alcohol is further metabolised in the liver. Approximately 2% of ester anaesthetics are excreted unchanged by the kidneys. The PABA analogues are responsible for the allergic reactions that frequently occur with the use of local anaesthetics of the ester type (see Section 10.5).

Anaesthetics of the amide type are metabolised in the liver first by the cytochrome P_{450} system. This reaction is followed by conjugation, resulting in highly water-soluble metabolites that are excreted by the kidneys. Between 70 and 90% of the amide anaesthetic is metabolised, and 10–30% is excreted by the kidneys unchanged.

The velocity of degradation in the liver is reciprocally related to the toxicity. Prilocaine is metabolised fastest and is consequently the least toxic amide-type local anaesthetic. Patients with severe liver insufficiency degrade amide-type local anaesthetics at a delayed rate, which increases the risk of a toxic effect (see Section 11.6).

3.4　　**Additives to local anaesthetics**

In addition to hydrochloric acid, to make the base form of local anaesthetic water soluble, several other ingredients are added to the solutions of the various local anaesthetics. The most important additives are vasoconstrictors and preservatives.

3.4.1　　Vasoconstrictors

Vasoconstrictors are extremely important in the clinical use of local anaesthetics. Without these compounds, the clinical use of local anaesthetics in dentistry would be hampered by their limited duration of action, as most anaesthetics produce vasodilatation. Exceptions are mepivacaine and prilocaine. Vasoconstrictors reduce the blood flow at the site of injection, which reduces the spread and resorption of the local anaesthetic, thereby enhancing the duration and intensity. In addition, vasoconstriction delays the absorption, which decreases systemic toxicity. Therefore, the vasoconstrictors adrenaline (also known as epinephrine) and felypressin are added to the local anaesthetics used in dentistry.

Adrenaline is an endogenous compound, released into the blood by the adrenal medulla, with a half-life of only a few minutes. Nervous or anxious people may have increased blood levels of adrenaline from fear of dental treatment. Vasoconstriction by adrenaline is achieved by stimulation of α_1-adrenergic receptors of the smooth muscles of the vessel wall. The maximum dose of adrenaline for adults is 200 µg.

Felypressin (octapressin) is a synthetic vasoconstrictor, derived from vasopressin (antidiuretic hormone). The vasoconstrictive activity of felypressin mainly originates from inducing constriction of the venous part of the circulation. The duration of action is longer than that of adrenaline. For adults, the maximum dose of felypressin is 5.4 µg.

The use of vasoconstrictors can have negative effects, both locally and systemically. The reduced blood flow decreases the pH of the tissue, which shifts the equilibrium reaction towards the ionised form of the anaesthetic. This reduces the penetration of the local anaesthetic in the nerve and diminishes the anaesthetic effect. In addition, decreased blood flow may have a negative effect on wound healing. A third local disadvantage is that a 'rebound' effect may occur as soon as the vasoconstrictor has worn off, due to the accumulation of degradation products; because of increased blood flow, there is an increased risk of secondary haemorrhage. After intravasal injection of an adrenaline-containing local anaesthetic, blood pressure and heart frequency will increase (dangerously).

3.4.2　　Preservatives

Methyl- and propylparaben are antibacterial agents (1 mg/ml). Because of their chemical structure, closely related to PABA, they frequently induce allergic reactions. Therefore, these preservatives are currently hardly ever added to local anaesthetic solutions.

Another preservative is bisulphite (0.3–2.0 mg/ml). This antioxidant is necessary to prevent oxidation of the vasoconstrictor potentially present, usually adrenaline. However, not only does bisulphite decrease the pH of the solution, but also some individuals may develop an allergy to this antioxidant.

3.5 Additives to topical anaesthetics

In the case of topical anaesthesia, a relatively highly concentrated solution of local anaesthetic is applied to the mucosa. The anaesthetic penetrates the surface tissue and the subsequent resorption can occur very rapidly. Topical anaesthesia is therefore characterised by the rapid onset (2 min) and short length (10 min) of anaesthesia. For dental practice, topical anaesthetics are available in the form of spray, gel and ointment.

Disadvantages of lidocaine-containing, alcohol-based spray are the rapid spread of the fluid over the mucosa and the very unpleasant taste. To reduce the unpleasant taste, flavouring substances such as banana essence, menthol and saccharin are added. In addition, polyethylene glycol is incorporated as a modifying agent. Direct administration of the spray to the mucosa shows a very high degree of absorption. For example, ten puffs of a lidocaine spray 10% are almost equivalent to an intravenous injection of 100 mg. Another disadvantage of using a spray is that it can cause irritation of the mucosa, especially of the oropharynx, probably induced by parabenes added to sprays as preservatives.

In the gel form, lidocaine is present as chloride, with methyl- and propylhydroxybenzoate as preservatives. By application of a gel at the injection site, the dose of topical anaesthetic can be kept very low and local. Sometimes patients with aphthous ulcers apply lidocaine gel before eating, enabling them to eat normally.

In ointments, lidocaine is present as a base, with polyethylene and propylene glycol added as modifying agents. The ointment also contains cellulose derivatives to improve the attachment to the oral mucosa. No further additives are present, but the possibility exists to add essences to improve the taste. Only a limited amount of lidocaine ointment 5% is necessary to achieve an anaesthetic effect.

General practical aspects

J.A. Baart

In dentistry, local anaesthesia is often required to be able to treat patients. Local anaesthesia facilitates a painless treatment, so that the patient's comfort is maximal during the treatment and so that the dentist is able to work calmly, with concentration and precision. This benefits the end result and the way this is achieved. Local anaesthesia is also used for diagnostic purposes to identify the cause of pain in the face, using selective anaesthesia. It is also used to prevent short- or long-term postoperative pain.

4.1　Use of local anaesthetics

Local anaesthesia may be applied preventatively when the dentist expects that dental treatment will be uncomfortable or painful and/or if the patient cannot bear pain very well. In other cases the anaesthetic is only used once pain does actually occur and/or if the patient indicates that he/she is no longer able to bear the pain.

Depending on the experience of the dentist and his/her knowledge of the patient's character, there is usually a preference for using preventative anaesthesia. This helps to increase the patient's confidence in the dentist and the treatment ('rather proactive than reactive'). Of course it makes a difference whether local anaesthesia is used for sub- or supragingival cleaning, for a cavity preparation, a crown or operative extraction of a wisdom tooth, or an extensive periodontal 'flap' procedure. There is also a difference in the way local anaesthetics are used for adults and children (see Chapter 8). Table 4.1 provides some general guidelines for the use of various techniques and indications for local anaesthesia.

4.2　Indications and contraindications

Before administration of an anaesthetic, the dentist must first explain why it is necessary. Indications and contraindications only have reference to the individual patient. Therefore, careful consideration must be made in the case of each patient, whether or not it is possible or suitable to use

Table 4.1	General guidelines and indications for the use of various techniques to administer local anaesthesia.	
Therapeutic/diagnostic	Lower jaw	Upper jaw
Cleaning		
Limited	INF	INF
Extensive	MB	INF
Filling/crown	MB + INF	INF
Endodontics	MB (IL)	INF
Extraction	MB + INF	INF
Periodontal surgery	MB + INF	HTA, INA, PN
M_3 inferior/superior extraction	MB + INF	NNP
Implantation	MB + INF	HTA + PN
Pre-implantological surgery	MB + MNB	HTA + PN
Central or peripheral pain?	MB	HTA + PN + INF
Dentogenic or non-dentogenic?	MB	INA, HTA
Which tooth?	IL	IL or INF

Abbreviations:
HTA　= high tuberosity anaesthesia (block anaesthesia)
IL　　= intraligamental anaesthesia
INA　= infraorbital nerve anaesthesia
INF　= infiltration anaesthesia
MB　= mandibular block (block anaesthesia)
MNB = mental nerve block
NNP = nasopalatine nerve anaesthesia
PN　= (greater) palatine nerve block

anaesthesia. This involves obtaining a good medical history and making enquiries related to previous experiences with local anaesthesia. The medical history should be well structured, systematic and preferably in written form. Negative findings such as 'no medication', 'no allergies' and 'no bleeding tendency' must also be documented. When enquiring about earlier experiences, it is important to continue asking for details, e.g. what the patient means by 'collapse' or 'allergy to adrenaline'. Some physical reactions may be based on a nervous, mostly involuntary response.

Examples of this are dizziness, nausea, stomach pains, fainting and sweating. Other symptoms, however, may indicate an overdose, allergic reactions or interaction with the prescribed medication that the patient is already taking. Table 11.1 gives recommendations for the use of local anaesthetics in medically compromised patients.

After explaining the nature of the anaesthesia, the dentist must verify whether the patient has understood this explanation. The patient may have additional questions that have to be answered first. Eventually the dentist will ask, more or less explicitly, for permission to anaesthetise (informed consent). If a patient does not protest against the use of a local anaesthetic, this does not mean that he/she is giving implicit permission (see Chapter 12).

4.3 Instruments

For the application of local anaesthetics in dentistry, almost exclusively use is made of glass cartridges with anaesthetic fluid, disposable needles and an aspirating syringe.

4.3.1 Cartridges

The glass cartridges usually contain 1.7–1.8 ml of anaesthetic fluid, although in the UK also 2.2 ml cartridges are available. In this textbook, recommendations are based on cartridges of 1.8 ml. The cartridge is closed, on one side by a rubber or synthetic diaphragm and on the other side by a rubber or synthetic stopper that may or may not be prepared for aspiration (Figure 4.1). The outside of the cartridge is printed with the name, composition and vasoconstrictor of the local anaesthetic. This information is printed on the glass or on a thin plastic foil. The latter ensures that, if the glass breaks (with intraligamental anaesthesia), the fragments are held together by the plastic foil and do not end up in the oral cavity (Figure 4.2).

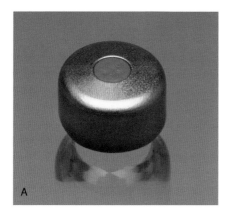

A

Figure 4.1 A
Top of an anaesthetic cartridge with diaphragm, into which the needle can be pierced.

Figure 4.1 B and C
Bottom of an anaesthetic
cartridge with stopper that
is (**B**) or is not (**C**) prepared
for aspiration.

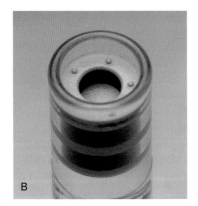

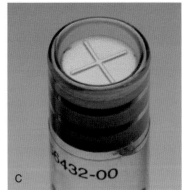

Figure 4.2 A and B
Glass anaesthetic cartridges
with plastic foil on which the
composition of the content
is noted; articaine 4% with
epinephrine 1:100,000
(**A**) and prilocaine 3% with
octapressin (**B**).

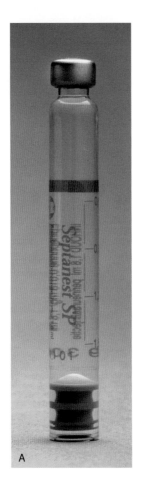

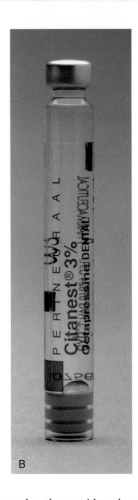

Cartridges are delivered in sterile packing and on the cartridges the expiry
date, the stock number and other information are written (Figure 4.3).
A cartridge that has just been unpacked does not need to be disinfected
before use with, for example, chlorhexidine in alcohol. It is also not
advisable, for various reasons, to preserve cartridges in disinfectant fluid.

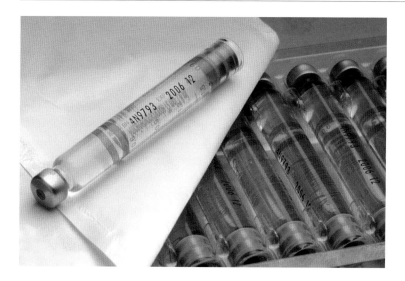

Figure 4.3
Cartridges are delivered in a sterile packing, and are printed with the stock number and expiry date.

The packs of cartridges can be kept at room temperature or in a fridge. If kept in a fridge, they must be taken out in plenty of time before use and – preferably – have reached body temperature. Having a cold anaesthetic fluid injected is particularly painful.

4.3.2   Needles

All needles used for local anaesthesia in dentistry are disposable and meant for single use only. The length of the needle is given in millimetres. A long needle is approx. 36 mm, a short one approx. 25 mm and an extra short needle is approx. 12 mm. These needles are suitable for regional block anaesthesia, infiltration anaesthesia and intraligamental anaesthesia respectively (Figure 4.4A). The diameter of the needle is measured in terms of gauge. The smaller the gauge number the larger the needle's diameter. Most needles used in dentistry have a gauge of 25–30. A number higher than 30 (i.e. very thin) should not be used, because aspiration of blood is then no longer possible. It is a misunderstanding that thinner needles are less painful than wider ones. It is primarily the needle pressure, the outflow speed of the liquid, the temperature and the pH that determine how painful an injection is. Reducing the needle diameter means that, with equal pressure, the liquid will be injected faster. Currently, so-called thin wall needles are in use, which have a wider lumen than the conventional needle.

The needle is contained in a metal or plastic cover. Part of the needle sticks out at the bottom and is meant to be inserted through the diaphragm into the anaesthetic fluid. The other part of the needle is used to actually apply the injection. The needles are packed in sterile packing and have two plastic caps that are removed from the needle by unscrewing and simultaneously bending them slightly (Figure 4.4B). After use the

Figure 4.4 A
Different types of injection
needles for local anaesthesia.
From top to bottom:
intraligamental needle,
short needle for infiltration
anaesthesia, longer needle for
block anaesthesia (e.g. for a
mandibular block) and a 'thin
wall needle' for block
anaesthesia.

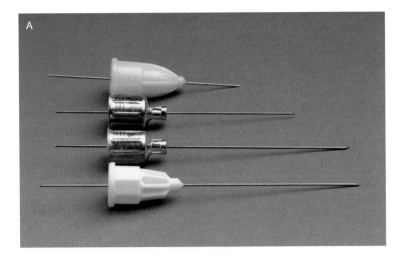

Figure 4.4 B
Removal of the back of the
disposable needle with a
turning and bending motion.

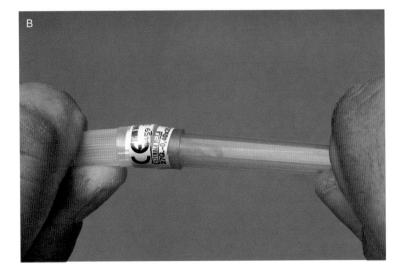

needle should be preferably completely disassembled and disposed of in
a sharps container. If such a container is not available, the cap should be
replaced carefully over the needle.

The needle is particularly flexible and can bend easily during mandibular
anaesthesia. This does not, however, cause the needle to break. Sometimes
it is necessary to bend the needle a little before injecting. This is the case,
for example, with anaesthesia in the floor of the mouth, in the palatine
canal and with high tuberosity anaesthesia. Even here the needle will not
break. Repetitive bending of the needle may, however, lead to breakage,
which is a serious complication (see Section 9.1).

4.3.3 The syringe

The cartridge syringe can usually be sterilised and is therefore made of rust-proof steel. Chromed steel is not advisable. Some cartridge syringes are made of plastic and thus disposable. There are two different types of syringes: an insert type and a snap-in type (see Figure 4.5).

The front of the cartridge syringe has screw thread into which the mantle of the needle can be screwed. The back of the syringe has a ring to facilitate aspiration. The syringe plunger must be linked to the stopper of the glass cartridge with anaesthetic fluid. This can be done in a variety of ways. Sometimes there is a little harpoon or spiral corkscrew that pierces the stopper. Other possibilities are a little cap or a blunt offset bulb that

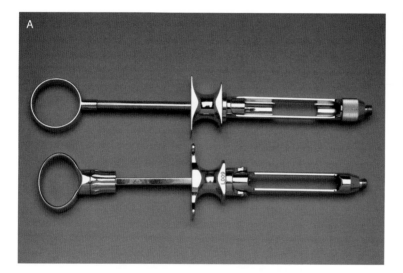

Figure 4.5 A
Cartridge syringes of rust-proof steel, insert type (above) and snap-in type (below).

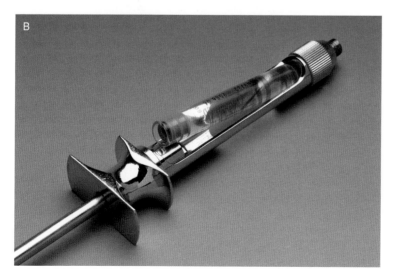

Figure 4.5 B
An insert-type syringe. By pulling back the plunger, the cartridge is laid into its place in the syringe.

Figure 4.5 C
A snap-in-type syringe. The cartridge can be placed in the syringe, once the plunger is slightly pulled back and the syringe is snapped open.

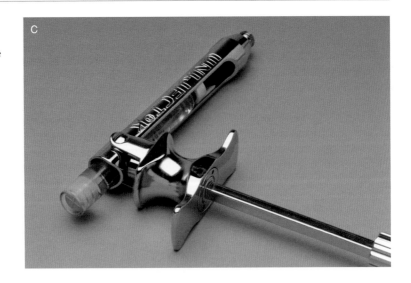

Figure 4.5 D1
The various parts of a ready-to-use syringe.

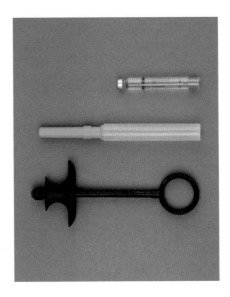

Figure 4.5 D2
A ready-to-use syringe after the administration of the local anaesthetic. Please note that the safety sleeve that initially covered the cartridge has now slid over the needle, which reduces the risk of needle stick accidents to almost zero.

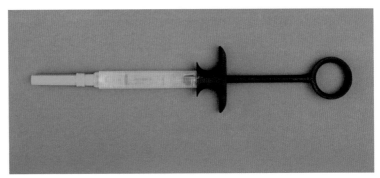

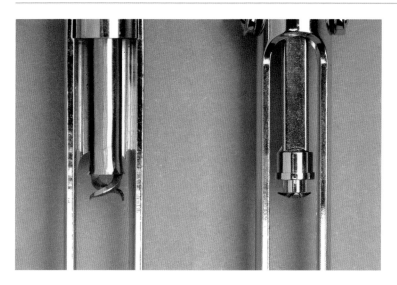

Figure 4.6
Cartridge syringes with corkscrew (left) at the end of the plunger and a little cap (right).

fits into a prepared opening at the back of the cartridge's stopper (see Figure 4.6).

Both the insert-type and snap-in-type syringes have a spring mechanism that aids automatic aspiration. By decreasing the pressure on the plunger, a few microlitres are sucked into the syringe, so it is easy to see whether the point of the needle is intravasal (Figure 4.7).

To prepare the cartridge syringe, the following steps are taken. First, a cartridge is placed in the syringe by pulling the plunger back slightly (insert type) or snapping it into the syringe (snap-in type). Then the plunger with harpoon, corkscrew, cap or bulb is pressed into the back of the rubber stopper to enable aspiration. After this, the mantle of the needle is screwed onto the screw thread of the front of the syringe. By applying slight pressure, one can now verify whether the syringe is ready to be used.

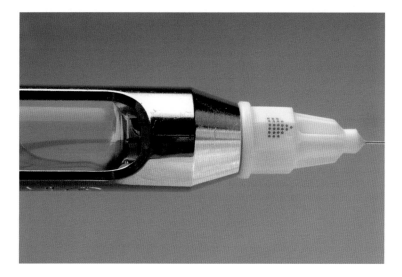

Figure 4.7
A cartridge syringe with a trace of blood visible in the cartridge after aspiration.

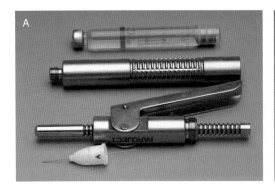
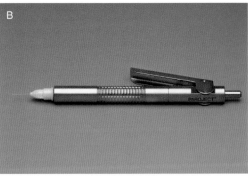

Figure 4.8 A and B
Intraligamental syringe;
disassembled (**A**) and
assembled (**B**). Light pressure
on the handle enables a
strong and uniform outflow
of the anaesthetic fluid. The
metal cover protects the glass
cartridge from breakage.

Once the first cartridge of anaesthetic fluid has been injected, it is possible that another cartridge will need to be applied, for example in another part of the patient's mouth. The plunger is disconnected from the back of the rubber stopper and pulled back completely. The cartridge can then be taken out and replaced by a new one. Once this is done the plunger with harpoon, corkscrew, cap or bulb is carefully reinserted into the back of the rubber stopper. This must be done *before* the syringe is checked for use because otherwise anaesthetic fluid will have leaked out of the needle already.

If during aspiration blood appears in the anaesthetic fluid, the cartridge must be replaced to ensure that when aspirating again there is no risk of the injection being given intravasally.

A combination of needle, cartridge and syringe is reserved for one patient only. In order to avoid confusion this combination must, therefore, be prepared per patient and not in advance.

Syringes for intraligamental anaesthesia have a deviant form. Intraligamental anaesthesia requires high pressure, which increases the risk of breaking the glass cartridge. Figure 4.8 shows an example of an intraligamental syringe. The plunger is moved forwards with a pumping motion. The cartridge is protected against breakage or its consequences, as it is completely surrounded by metal. In order to prevent ischaemic damage to the periodontal ligament as a result of the fluid pressure and/or vasoconstrictor, it is advisable to wait briefly between each pumping motion. Intraligamental anaesthesia applied with a microprocessor-controlled pump (the Wand®) does not present this problem, since the outflow speed is very low (see Figure 8.10).

4.4   Topical anaesthesia

Occasionally it is advisable to apply preliminary anaesthesia. The benefits lie partly in the anaesthesia of the point of injection and partly in psychological factors. Preliminary anaesthesia for intraligamental and block anaesthesia has a limited effect and is therefore not advocated. Preliminary anaesthesia may be beneficial for infiltration anaesthesia (Figure 4.9).

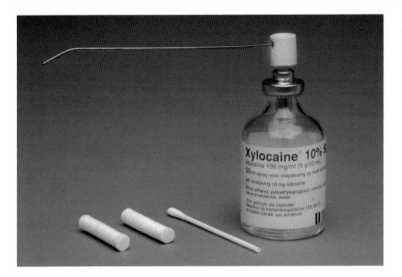

Figure 4.9
Topical anaesthesia with
use of lidocaine spray 10%.
Application is carried out
with a roll of cotton wool
or a cotton bud.

In contrast to what is stated in the accompanying guidelines, it is better
not to use anaesthetic spray directly in the mouth. Lidocaine spray 10%
is very easily absorbed by the mucosa of the oral–throat cavity, which
increases the risk of children being overdosed. Moreover, the spray nozzle
must be cleaned and sterilised again, even after a single use. It is therefore
better to apply the spray fluid or anaesthetic gel to a roll of cotton wool or
the tip of a cotton bud. This allows the dentist, the dental assistant or
patients themselves to apply a very precise preliminary anaesthesia. It is
enough to apply the spray fluid or gel 2–3 minutes before inserting the
injection needle (Box 4.1).

Box 4.1

Topical anaesthesia without subsequent infiltration or block anaesthesia
is not enough for dental treatment, since the depth and duration of
topical anaesthesia are limited.

4.5   **Position of the patient and dentist**

In dentistry, local anaesthetics are often applied preventatively, i.e. before
any pain occurs due to the treatment. Some dentists therefore anaesthetise
patients while they are sitting up in the dentist's chair. This is not right.
The view into the mouth is not optimal, the position of the lamp is not
ideal and, in case of a vasovagal collapse (see Section 10.2), the patient may
fall off the chair forwards. It is therefore sensible to apply local anaesthesia
with the dentist and patient in the same position they have during the
subsequent treatment. This means that usually the patient is

Figure 4.10
The dentist holds the head of
the patient steady with the
non-injecting hand.

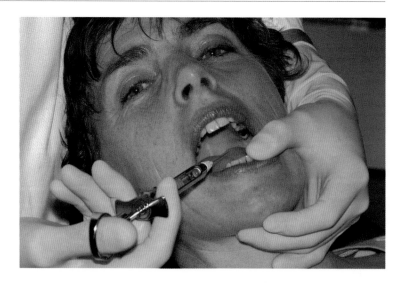

Figure 4.10
The dentist holds the head of the patient steady with the non-injecting hand.

anaesthetised in a semi-horizontal to horizontal position. The dentist sits next to the dental chair in a 9–1 o'clock position, while the assistant sits in a 2–3 o'clock position.

During administration of the anaesthetic, the dentist should hold the patient's head steady with the arm and free non-injecting hand (Figure 4.10). Any unexpected movement of the patient will then not lead to self-injury or injection in the wrong place. Moreover, especially with mandibular block anaesthesia and infraorbital nerve anaesthesia, it is easier to find the point of injection with the steadying and feeling hand. The possibility of the dentist pricking his/her own hand if the patient's head moves unexpectedly is very slight and not unduly dangerous for the dentist's health if it happens with an unused needle. Nevertheless, some dentists have a dental mirror or wooden spatula in the non-injecting hand to protect themselves from self-injection.

Just before the needle actually penetrates the mucosa, the mucosa is stretched and, if possible, the dentist carefully pinches the patient's lip or cheek to mask the prick. An intravasal injection is avoided by aspirating before injecting and repeating this after every change of position of the needle. The injection itself must be given very slowly. The injection speed may be a little higher for free mucosa. The dentist must continually ask for the patient's experience of the local anaesthesia both during and directly after the injection. Young and nervous patients should be given compliments for the way they handled the anaesthesia.

It is not correct to anaesthetise a patient and then ask him/her to sit in the waiting room until the anaesthesia has taken effect. Local anaesthesia takes effect in between 30 and 180 seconds and this does not justify leaving a recently anaesthetised patient in the waiting room without proper supervision. During or immediately after an injection unexpected reactions may occur.

If the patient has an undesired reaction during or after applying a local anaesthetic, the dentist must react calmly. It is important that the dentist gives a good explanation and, if necessary, an apology. For example, a patient could experience palpitations after an intravascular injection with a local anaesthetic containing adrenaline. 'Blanching' may appear in the face. In this case a comforting explanation will suffice. If a nerve is pricked, e.g. the inferior alveolar nerve, lingual nerve or mental nerve, the patient will need more than an explanation and calming word. In this case the feeling may be altered for days, weeks and sometimes months (see Chapter 9).

Undesired reactions to local anaesthesia may, of course, also be related to the dentist's skill and injection method. Assembling the anaesthetic syringe in front of the patient and checking whether the anaesthetic fluid is ready by ostentatiously tapping the syringe and holding it to the ceiling to release any air bubbles will not reassure the average patient. A sudden or rough application of a local anaesthetic must be avoided. The injection must be given extremely slowly anywhere in the mouth and especially in the palatal mucosa.

4.6   Verification of effectiveness

To verify the effectiveness of the anaesthesia, the dentist should first ask the patient open questions: 'Do you feel any change yet? What do you feel? Could you indicate where it is tingling or where it feels numb?' If the patient's answers are unclear, the dentist can help the patient by asking: 'What about the lip? And the tongue?' If necessary, he/she can ask about differences in feeling: 'Does it have the same feeling as this side? If I touch here, does it feel the same as there?' The dentist must avoid asking closed questions that can be answered with a 'yes' or 'no' because the answers are unreliable. 'Is the lip tingling already? And the tongue?' must not be asked after anaesthesia. Some combinations of anaesthesia may lead to incorrect information from the patient about the effects of the local anaesthesia. If mandibular block anaesthesia is directly followed by infiltration anaesthesia in the lower jaw's premolar area, a one-sided numbed lower lip does not say much. Therefore, it is better in these cases to give the mandibular block first, to wait for a more or less spontaneous reaction from the patient, who may say the lower lip has begun to tingle, and only then to continue with infiltration anaesthesia buccal to the lower premolars.

It is proper practice towards the patient to give a little prick with, for example, a dental probe to test the anaesthesia before proceeding to the painful treatment. An ineffective anaesthesia that is not noticed by the dentist, followed by a painful treatment, damages the patient's confidence in the dentist and his/her treatment. In certain cases the dentist might use additional techniques such as suggestive relaxation, hypnosis and inhalation sedatives. Some patients may also be given medication that relaxes or makes them drowsy, or general anaesthesia, which is usually given intravenously.

5 Local anaesthesia in the upper jaw

J.A. Baart

5.1 Introduction

Sensory innervation of the upper jaw arises from the second trunk of the trigeminal nerve, the maxillary nerve. This main branch of the trigeminal nerve leaves the neurocranium via the foramen rotundum, reaches the pterygopalatine fossa and runs straight through as the infraorbital nerve, branching off many times along its course. With regard to local anaesthesia in the upper jaw, the following branches are of importance:
- the greater and lesser palatine nerves;
- the posterior, middle and anterior superior alveolar nerves;
- the infraorbital nerve (Figure 5.1).

Figure 5.1

The course of the maxillary nerve and its main branches.

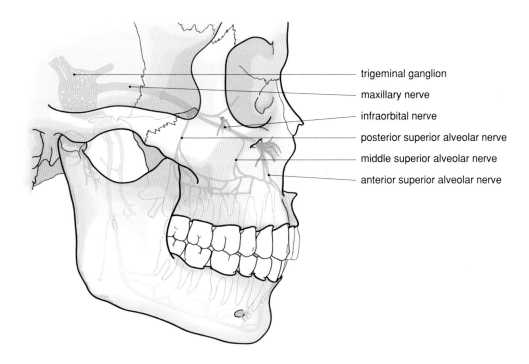

- trigeminal ganglion
- maxillary nerve
- infraorbital nerve
- posterior superior alveolar nerve
- middle superior alveolar nerve
- anterior superior alveolar nerve

Thus the main trunk of the maxillary nerve can be reached via the greater palatine foramen, via the infraorbital foramen as well as from high behind the maxillary tuberosity. In practice, high tuberosity anaesthesia is the only practical regional block anaesthesia for almost the entire maxillary nerve. Therefore this regional block anaesthesia technique is used for surgical procedures.

For everyday dental procedures in the upper jaw, infiltration anaesthesia is commonly used. The cortical bone of the outer surface of the upper jaw is relatively thin, which facilitates the diffusion of local anaesthetic fluid. All (buccal) roots of the upper teeth can be reached in this way. The palatine roots of the molars and possibly the premolars are anaesthetised by infiltration anaesthesia of the branches of the greater palatine nerve and those of the nasopalatine nerve. Regional block anaesthesia is also possible via the greater palatine foramen and the nasopalatine canal.

Infiltration anaesthesia of the upper jaw is particularly effective, unless an injection is made into an inflamed area. Regional block anaesthesia of the greater palatine, nasopalatine and infraorbital nerves is equally effective. In cases of regional block anaesthesia using a high tuberosity block, it is usually only the posterior superior alveolar and medial branches that are numbed, but sometimes also the palatine and infraorbital nerves.

5.2 Incisors and canines

5.2.1 Anatomical aspects

Before leaving the infraorbital foramen the infraorbital nerve branches off in the infraorbital canal towards the incisors and canines, the anterior superior alveolar nerves. These nerve branches provide the sensory innervation of the incisor and canine pulp, as well as the vestibular fold, the gingiva, the periosteum and the bone. They anastomose with small branches of the other vestibular side (Figure 5.2). The nasopalatine nerve leaves the incisive foramen, and provides the sensory innervation of the palatine bone, periosteum and mucosa (Figure 5.3). Because of the relatively thin and porous nature of the maxilla's cortical bone, an extraperiosteal (infiltration) anaesthetic can spread easily within the maxillary bone.

The apices of the root of the central incisor and canine are found on the buccal side of the bone, whilst the apex of the lateral incisor is found on the palatinal side. This must be taken into consideration when infiltration anaesthetics are given, especially when used for an apicoectomy. The anterior superior alveolar branches run from high lateral to low medial. For this reason, infiltration anaesthetics may best be applied laterally, just above the apex.

5.2.2 Indication

For cavity preparations in the upper frontal teeth, buccal or labial infiltration anaesthesia is usually sufficient. The same applies to

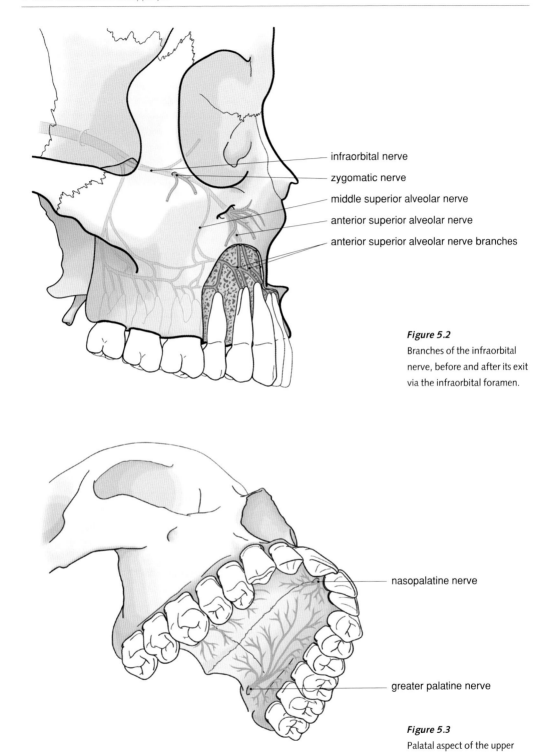

Figure 5.2
Branches of the infraorbital nerve, before and after its exit via the infraorbital foramen.

infraorbital nerve

zygomatic nerve

middle superior alveolar nerve

anterior superior alveolar nerve

anterior superior alveolar nerve branches

nasopalatine nerve

greater palatine nerve

Figure 5.3
Palatal aspect of the upper jaw with the nasopalatine and greater palatine nerves.

Figure 5.4
A cotton bud, soaked with a topical anaesthetic, in the nose of a patient in order to numb the intraossal branches of the nasopalatine nerve.

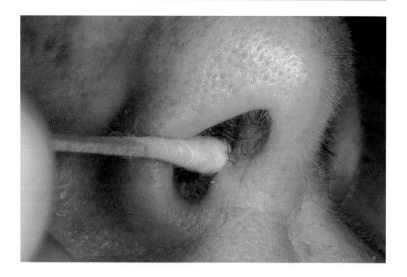

endodontic treatments. In cases where a cofferdam is used, or wedges, supplementary palatine anaesthesia is sometimes required. For crown preparations, it is sensible to use buccal and palatine infiltration anaesthesia.

For surgical procedures in the upper frontal teeth area, such as periodontal surgery, implants, extractions and apicoectomies, it is advisable to anaesthetise a larger area using regional block anaesthesia with supplementary infiltration anaesthesia. Because regional block anaesthesia is highly effective in this area, it can be directly followed by infiltration anaesthesia. The infraorbital and nasopalatine nerves can be reached via the infraorbital foramen and the nasopalatine canal. Infiltration anaesthesia is given in the buccal area and, if necessary, in the interdental (palatine) papillae. Nevertheless, there are exceptions where good anaesthesia is not achieved. The intraossal branches of the nasopalatine nerve are responsible for this. These smaller branches can be anaesthetised by an injection or the application of a cotton bud with anaesthetic ointment in the respective nostril (Figure 5.4).

5.2.3   Technique

Buccal infiltration anaesthesia of the upper frontal teeth is performed by lifting the lip with the free hand, gently pinching the lip and then piercing the mucosa of the buccal fold with the needle, just above the apex of the respective tooth. The syringe is thereby held parallel to the longitudinal axis of the tooth. The needle is inserted no more than 3–5 mm. Any contact of the needle point with the periosteum or the bone must be avoided, and the fluid must be injected slowly. Aspiration is recommended but not really necessary: there are no large blood vessels in this area (Figure 5.5).

Palatine infiltration anaesthesia is applied in the palatal gingiva of the respective tooth. This anaesthesia is particularly painful if the needle is

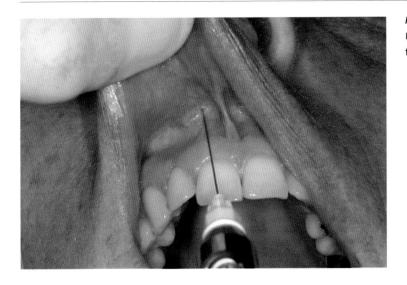

Figure 5.5
Infiltration anaesthesia for
the I$_1$ superior right.

moved up over the periosteum and when not injected extremely slowly. It is, therefore, sensible to insert the needle tangentially and not to move it up, or to resort to palatine conduction anaesthesia for the central and lateral incisors (Figure 5.6A and B).

There is usually enough space for an anaesthetic around the canines at the transition between the vertical and horizontal sections of the palate. Here the space for injection fluid is maximum sub- and supraperiostally. Here too it is necessary to inject extremely slowly.

The required amount of local anaesthetic is small, both for buccal and palatine anaesthesia. For buccal anaesthesia a quarter of a cartridge per tooth is sufficient, whereas a maximum of an eighth of a cartridge is needed for palatine anaesthesia. Sometimes it is necessary, in cases of periodontal or implant procedures, to inject anaesthetics into the interdental papillae, but this is painful for the patient. The dentist should, therefore, wait until the vestibular and/or palatine infiltration anaesthetic takes effect, before anaesthetising the interdental papillae.

See Section 7.2 for a description of the block anaesthesia of the greater palatine and infraorbital nerves.

Figure 5.6 A and B
Drawing (**A**) and photo (**B**) of regional block anaesthesia of the nasopalatine nerve. The needle is inserted at an angle into the incisive papilla to avoid damaging the nerve and bleeding from the vessels in the nasopalatine canal.

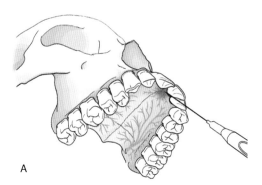

A

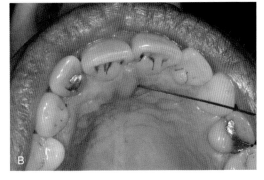

B

5.3   Premolars

5.3.1   Anatomical aspects

Sensory innervation of the first and second premolars in the upper jaw arises from the superior alveolar nerve, via the middle and anterior superior alveolar branches. The middle superior alveolar branches run from high dorsal to low ventral, whereas the anterior superior alveolar branches come from the upper frontal area (Figure 5.7).

Furthermore, because the lateral aspect of the upper jaw in this area is concave, the needle must be inserted a fraction from out to in, in order to inject close to the periosteum. The facial artery runs near the first premolar, high in the buccal fold, so aspiration prior to injection is indispensable.

Innervation of the premolar area arises on the palatal side from branches of the greater palatine nerve and also from smaller branches of the nasopalatine nerve that run dorsally (Figure 5.3).

Besides the branches of the greater palatine nerve, the greater palatine artery and vein also run along the palatinal side, at the transition from the vertical to the horizontal aspect. An intravasal injection must be avoided

Figure 5.7

The course of the superior alveolar nerve and of the middle and anterior superior alveolar branches.

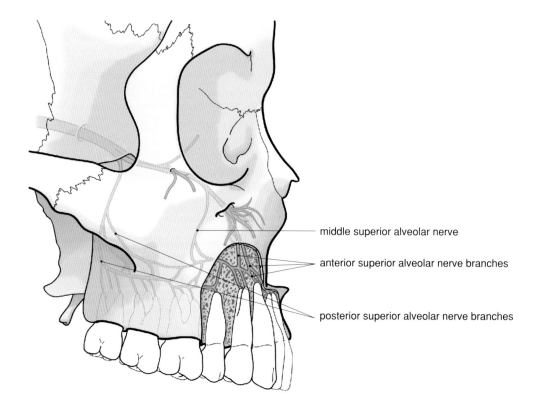

middle superior alveolar nerve

anterior superior alveolar nerve branches

posterior superior alveolar nerve branches

by careful aspiration. Piercing the artery here also has the disadvantage of causing persistent bleeding from the needle hole. On the other hand, the injection must not be too superficial, since a high injective pressure is then required, which will result in a lot of pain, and ischaemic necrosis of the palatal mucosa may occur after treatment (see Section 9.8).

5.3.2 Indication

Buccal infiltration anaesthesia is sufficient for cavity preparations and endodontic treatments. If the first premolar of the upper jaw (P_{1sup}) has two diverging roots, additional palatal anaesthesia may be needed. This supplementary palatal anaesthesia is also needed for crown preparations. For surgical operations, such as periodontal surgery, implantology, extraction and apicoectomy, a larger anaesthetised area is required. For this reason, the anaesthetic is injected into the vestibular area at a point much higher than the apices, and in the palatal area the anaesthetic is injected near the apices at the point of transition from the horizontal to the vertical aspect. Though palatine block anaesthesia is possible, it is discouraged as it requires two injections: one into the greater palatine foramen and another into the incisive papilla.

5.3.3 Technique

In the upper jaw the transversal width of the alveolar process is narrowest in the area of the canines and rapidly increases in a dorsal direction. The apices of the roots of the first premolar lie, when they are bi-rooted and divergent, immediately below the buccal and palatal cortical bone, respectively. The single-rooted second premolar has an apex that lies more centrally in the alveolar process. This must be kept in mind when a local anaesthetic is applied here.

The corner of the patient's mouth is lifted and the free hand should pinch the lip carefully, so that the needle's penetration into the buccal mucosa is hardly felt. With the point of the needle a small amount of anaesthetic fluid is deposited just above and dorsal to the apex (Figure 5.8A and B). Aspiration for injection near the first premolar must be carried out in order to avoid an intravasal injection. If the fluid is injected intravasally the patient will feel a short, sharp shot of pain in the face, and the skin of the cheek and lower eyelid will pale immediately (*blanching*).

The needle must be inserted from out to in. For restorative dental treatments the needle point should be approx. 5 mm above the apex. For surgical procedures a more cranial infiltration anaesthesia is required. On the palatal side, the needle is inserted counter-laterally and vertically at the transition of the horizontal to the vertical aspect of the palate (Figure 5.9). After aspiration, the fluid is injected extremely slowly. The amount of anaesthetic fluid used in the buccal area is approx. 1 ml and a maximum of 0.25 ml is used for the palatal side.

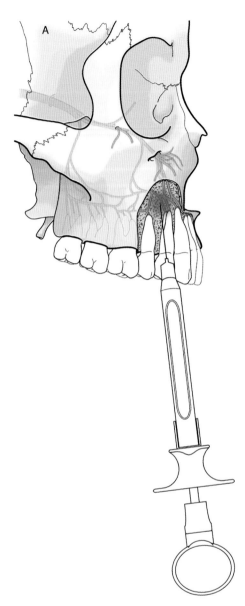

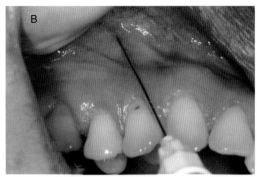

Figure 5.8 A and B
Drawing (**A**) and photo (**B**) of
the infiltration anaesthesia of
the P$_1$ superior right.

5.4   **Molars**

5.4.1   Anatomical aspects

The posterior superior alveolar branches innervate the buccal side of the
molar region of the upper jaw. The source of these branches of the second
trunk of the trigeminal nerve is high in the pterygopalatine fossa and they
run along the maxillary tuberosity to the low ventral area. They provide
sensitivity in the M$_3$, M$_2$ and M$_1$ and the mucosa, gingiva, periosteum

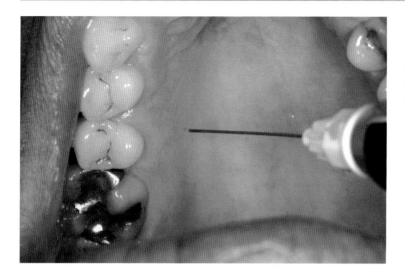

Figure 5.9
Palatine infiltration anaesthesia of the P_1 and P_2 superior right. The needle is inserted from the left into the transitional area of the horizontal to vertical sections of the palate.

and the bone (Figure 5.10). The palatal mucosa and palatal root of the first molar in the upper jaw (M_{1sup}) are innervated by the greater palatine nerve, which also comes from the second trunk of the trigeminal nerve (see Figure 5.3).

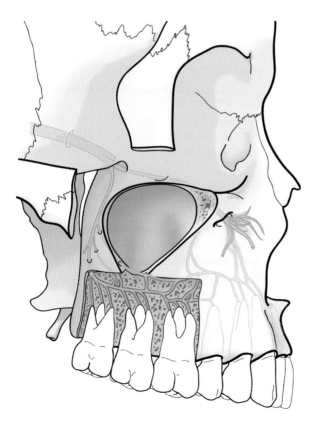

Figure 5.10
The course of the superior alveolar nerve and the posterior superior alveolar branches.

The zygomatic buttress is found in the buccal area above the apices of the M_{1sup}. The point of attachment can vary, however, so that an impermeable cortical layer of bone may sometimes be found lateral to the buccal roots of M_{1sup}, depending on the length of the vestibulary radices and the crest's point of attachment.

The position of the roots of the M_2 and the erupted M_{3sup} is more or less central in the bone, depending on the level of convergence. The transversal width of the alveolar process in the molar region is considerable, so that more anaesthetic fluid is needed for adequate numbing. The pterygoid venous plexus is found laterally high to the maxillary tuberosity.

5.4.2   Indication

For cavity preparations in the M_{1sup} both buccal and palatal infiltration anaesthesia is required. For the second and third molar in the upper jaw, vestibulary anaesthesia will suffice for these indications. The same applies with regard to endodontal treatment of this area. If the M_{1sup} happens to have long buccal roots and/or a low-positioned zygomatic buttress, the infiltration anaesthesia must be applied behind the crest, i.e. higher and more dorsal.

For operative treatments such as periodontal surgery, implantology, extraction or apicoectomy (of the buccal roots), regional block anaesthesia is commonly used high above the maxillary tuberosity and at the position of the greater palatine foramen, supplemented with some buccal infiltration anaesthesia. The method of high tuberosity anaesthesia is described in Section 7.1.1.

Regional block anaesthesia of the major palatine nerve is administered vertically from the counter-lateral corner of the mouth. The needle must not be inserted too deeply in the direction of the foramen in order to avoid damage to the nerve or piercing the artery. Aspiration prior to the actual injection is prescribed.

The amount of anaesthetic fluid for buccal infiltration anaesthesia should be approx. 1–1.5 ml. For palatine infiltration or block anaesthesia, no more than 0.25 ml is required.

Patients that are given an infiltration anaesthetic in the molar region of the upper jaw can have the impression that the anaesthetic has not worked. They compare the feeling they observe with the sensation that they know from an infiltration anaesthetic in the premolar region or the front teeth or from mandibular regional block anaesthesia. It is therefore wise to explain to patients this difference in sensation.

5.4.3   Technique

Infiltration anaesthesia on the buccal side of the upper molars is applied at an angle from the front. The jaw here is flat to convex. The zygomatic buttress sticks outwards and is found near the first molar. The point of the needle should be inserted right above and dorsal to the apices

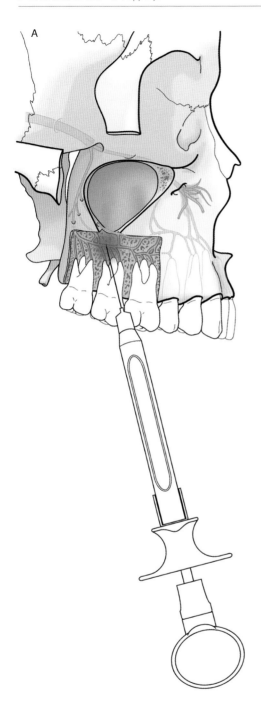

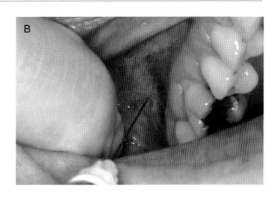

Figure 5.11 A and B

Drawing (**A**) and photo (**B**) of infiltration anaesthesia of the M_2 superior right. The needle is inserted slightly from out to in.

(Figure 5.11A and B). For the first molar it is occasionally necessary to inject behind the crest and slightly higher, due to the inaccessibility of the buccal roots through the thick cortical bone. For the palatal side, infiltration anaesthesia of the major palatine nerve at the first molar, and regional block anaesthesia for the second and third molar, are sufficient

A

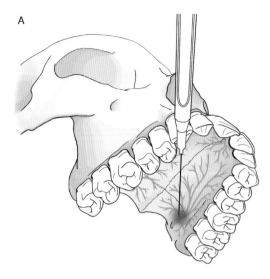

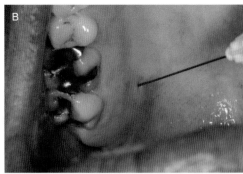

Figure 5.12 A and B

Drawing (**A**) and photo
(**B**) of the palatal regional
block anaesthesia of the
greater palatine nerve.
Careful aspiration prior to
injection is required!

(Figure 5.12A and B). For an extraction of the second and erupted third
molar, an injection of 0.25 ml fluid next to the gingival fold on the palatal
side will suffice (Figure 5.13). See Section 7.1.1. for a description of the high
tuberosity anaesthesia method.

Figure 5.13

Palatal infiltration anaesthesia
of the gingiva on the level of
the M_2 superior right.

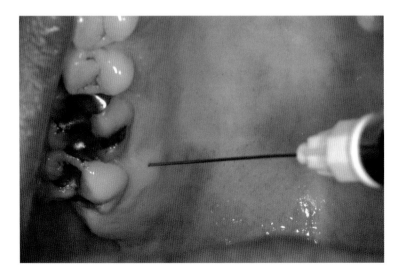

5.5 The impacted third molar of the upper jaw

5.5.1 Anatomical aspects

The impacted third molar of the upper jaw (M_{3sup}) is usually found completely in the maxillary tuberosity with a slight distovestibular inclination. Here, the buccal cortical bone is very thin. Slightly higher and in a more lateral position is the pterygoid venous plexus. The branches of the second trunk of the trigeminal nerve, and the maxillary artery and vein, run behind the tuberosity and higher in the pterygopalatine fossa. On the palatine side of the impacted M_{3sup} are the greater palatine foramen and the lesser palatine foramina, from which the palatine nerves branch off that innervate the palatine gingiva and the soft palate. The greater palatine arteries and vein also come from the greater palatine foramen. Therefore, the area lateral, dorsal and medial to the impacted M_{3sup} is richly innervated and vascularised. Here surgery outside of the periosteum is risky.

5.5.2 Indication

In dental practice, local anaesthesia will only be used in this area for the removal of an impacted M_{3sup} or for harvesting bone for pre-implant treatment elsewhere in the mouth.

5.5.3 Technique

Anaesthesia of the entire greater palatine nerve and, if necessary, of the lesser palatine nerves is performed with regional block anaesthesia. The needle is brought forwards from the counter-lateral corner of the mouth in the direction of the greater and lesser palatine foramens (Figure 5.12A and B). Touching the nerve or piercing the artery must be avoided. For this reason aspiration is necessary. Approximately 0.25 ml anaesthetic fluid is sufficient. Refer to Section 7.1.1 for information on the method of high maxillary tuberosity anaesthesia.

6 Local anaesthesia in the lower jaw

J.A. Baart

Introduction

The buccal cortical bone at the premolars and molars of the lower jaw impedes the diffusion of anaesthetic fluid to the apices of these teeth, located centrally in the jaw bone. Adults require mandibular block anaesthesia for an effective anaesthesia. In the area of the lower canines and incisors the cortical bone is thinner and the roots lie on the buccal side of the jaw. Here, infiltration anaesthesia is effective.

The mental nerve leaves the jaw through the mental foramen and innervates the buccal mucosa and gingiva, the lower lip and the skin of the chin. Therefore, anaesthetising the mental nerve will not anaesthetise the teeth in adults. However, in children the molars are anaesthetised, because the apex of these teeth is reached through diffusion through the thinner cortical bone.

The lingual side of the mandible is innervated by the lingual nerve. This nerve can be anaesthetised both by block anaesthesia as well as by infiltration anaesthesia. The dentist must avoid pricking the floor of the mouth too often as this increases the risk of a haematoma in combination with transport of bacteria via the injection needle. This may cause a phlegmonous infection of the mouth floor, a life-threatening complication.

Block anaesthesia of the buccal nerve is possible. This nerve runs from high lingual and crosses the front side of the mandibular ramus above the occlusion plane. Then the buccal nerve continues caudo-ventrally to innervate the buccal mucosa and gingiva in the area of the (erupted) M_{3inf} to P_{2inf}. Because the height at which the buccal nerve crosses the mandibula varies, infiltration anaesthesia applied buccal to the respective teeth is also an excellent technique to anaesthetise the gingiva and mucosa (Figures 6.1 and 6.2).

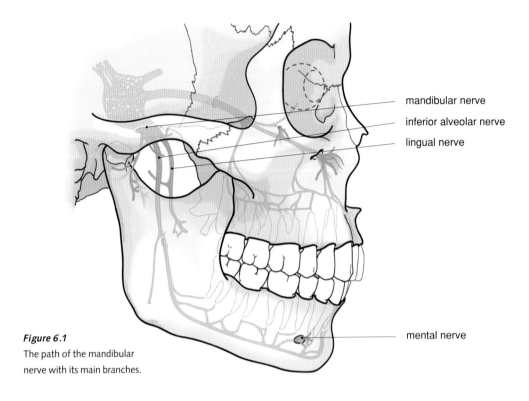

Figure 6.1
The path of the mandibular
nerve with its main branches.

mandibular nerve

inferior alveolar nerve

lingual nerve

mental nerve

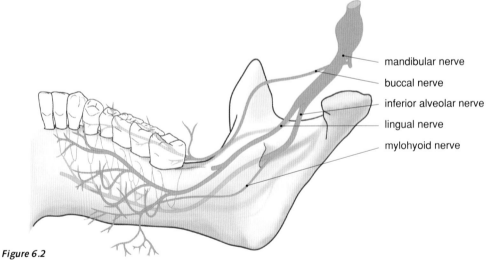

Figure 6.2
Medial aspect of the path of
the mandibular nerve and its
branches: the buccal nerve,
lingual nerve and inferior
alveolar nerve.

mandibular nerve

buccal nerve

inferior alveolar nerve

lingual nerve

mylohyoid nerve

6.2 Incisors and canines

6.2.1 Anatomical aspects

Once the alveolar nerve has separated from the trigeminal nerve, the nerve runs laterally and enters the mandibular foramen. The inferior alveolar nerve divides into a branch, the mental nerve, at the mental foramen and then continues as the incisive nerve. The incisive nerve no longer runs in a bony canal and divides into little branches leading to the roots of the lower canines and incisors (Figure 6.3). In the mandibular symphysis area, sensory anastomoses from the contralateral side are present, both lingually and buccally. This must be taken into account, particularly with extensive surgical treatment in the lower frontal area.

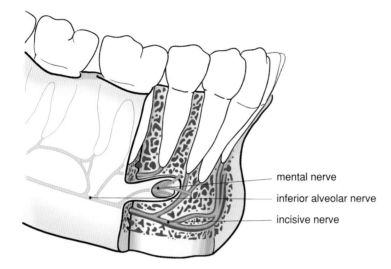

mental nerve

inferior alveolar nerve

incisive nerve

Figure 6.3
The path of the mental and incisive nerves.

The roots of the lower incisors and canines are found against the buccal cortical bone. The mental muscle is attached to the jaw at the height of the I_{2inf} so that infiltration anaesthesia in this area can be painful and less effective.

6.2.2 Indication

Buccal infiltration anaesthesia will be sufficient for cavity preparations and endodontic treatment in the lower frontal area, unless a cofferdam and/or matrix band and wedges are used. In that case, it is necessary to apply additional anaesthesia lingually, or perhaps in the interdental papilla on the lingual side.

Infiltration anaesthesia is also used for surgical treatment in the lower frontal area, in which case the needle is inserted more caudally to the apex. The dentist must take the sensory anastamoses into account by also

Figure 6.4 A and B
Drawing (**A**) and photo (**B**) of infiltration anaesthesia of the I_2 inferior right. The buccal gingiva is also anaesthetised. In order to anaesthetise the lingual gingiva, it is necessary to inject into the floor of the mouth.

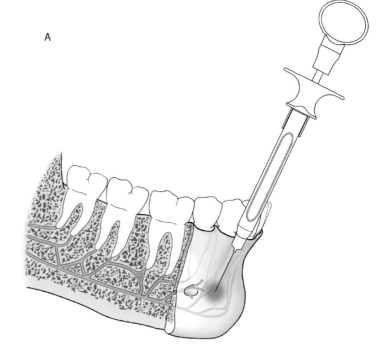

A

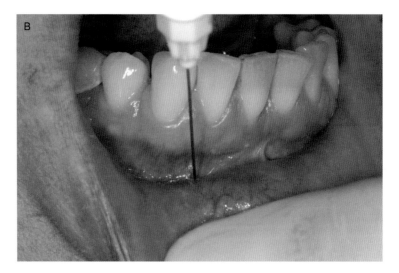

B

anaesthetising the contralateral nerve branches. The point of attachment of the mimic muscles, such as the orbicularis oris muscle and the mental muscle, also requires special attention during anaesthesia. Injecting into these muscles causes bleeding, is painful and does not lead to a good anaesthesia.

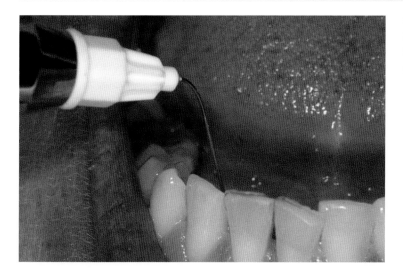

Figure 6.4 C Lingual anaesthesia with a bent needle with the dentist in an 8 to 9 o'clock position.

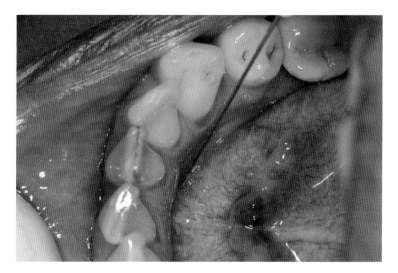

Figure 6.4 D Lingual anaesthesia with a non-bent needle with the dentist in an 11 to 1 o'clock position.

6.2.3 Technique

For infiltration anaesthesia in the lower frontal area, the non-injecting hand pulls the lip forwards and pinches the lip softly at the moment the needle penetrates the mucosa. The needle is inserted right under the apex of the tooth that is to be anaesthetised, up to the bone. Preferably, the needle is inserted vertically and not pushed into the periosteum. The dentist sits or stands behind the patient in an 11–1 o'clock position. The same position is assumed for infiltration anaesthesia of the lingual mucosa and gingiva. When anaesthetising from an 8–9 o'clock position, it is better to bend the needle 45–90 degrees for a lingual injection (Figure 6.4), but a disadvantage of this is that the needle cannot be returned to its protective cap. With lingual anaesthesia it is important to prevent a haematoma occurring.

Bilateral mandibular block anaesthesia, with additional local infiltration anaesthesia, is recommended for surgical treatment of the lower front, such as extensive pre-implantological treatments (e.g. a chin bone transplant) and implantological treatments (two or four dental implants). This reduces the required number of injections to a minimum, as well as the chance of haematomas and infections. Furthermore, a maximum of 4–6 ml of anaesthetic fluid will be sufficient.

In this situation it is recommended that the dentist administers the double-sided mandibular block first and then waits until the patient spontaneously indicates that the lower lip and border of the tongue have started to tingle. The dentist can then give a buccal infiltration anaesthesia.

6.3 Premolars

6.3.1 Anatomical aspects

Innervation of the premolars in the lower jaw takes place in the bone through the inferior alveolar nerve, buccal through the buccal nerve (at the P_{1inf} also through the mental nerve) and lingually through the lingual nerve. Because of the thickness and impermeability of the buccal cortical bone, infiltration anaesthesia is not really possible for the treatment of the (pulpa of) premolars in adult patients.

Use of block anaesthesia of the mandibular nerve, i.e. of the inferior alveolar and lingual nerves, is therefore a more obvious choice, if necessary supplemented with local infiltration anaesthesia of the branches of the buccal nerve (Figure 6.5). The mental nerve is found lower than the apices, exactly between the two premolars. Block anaesthesia of the mental nerve branches must be given superficially to avoid damage to the mental nerve, with subsequent long-term anaesthesia of the lower lip half.

If a combination of block anaesthesia of the mandibular nerve and local infiltration is chosen, then the mandibular block must, of course, be given first. A supplementary infiltration anaesthetic is applied locally once the patient spontaneously reports that the lower lip half and edge of the tongue have begun to tingle. When the inferior alveolar nerve appears to be anaesthetised after block anaesthesia of the mandibular nerve, but the lingual nerve does not, then lingual infiltration anaesthesia at the level of the respective premolar will be sufficient. Generally, a repeated mandibular block injection should be avoided, because the partial anaesthesia that has already set in will limit the patient's ability to give a warning if the lingual or inferior alveolar nerve is touched by the needle.

6.3.2 Indication

Mandibular block anaesthesia is used for cavity preparation and endodontic treatment, if necessary supplemented by buccal infiltration anaesthesia (Figure 6.6). It should also be used for extensive surgical

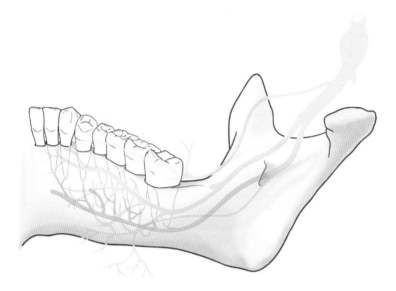

Figure 6.5
The path of the branches of the mandibular nerve in the premolar area.

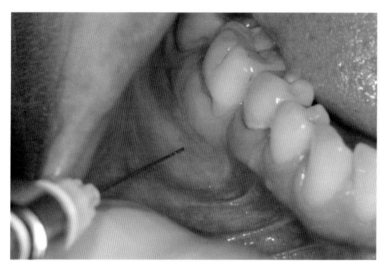

Figure 6.6
Buccal infiltration anaesthesia at the level of the M_1 inferior right, for anaesthetising the buccal nerve branches.

treatments such as periodontal surgery, implantology, extraction and apicoectomy, where the buccal infiltration anaesthesia is more extensive and more caudal. Extra attention to the path of the mental nerve is required here. When giving additional anaesthesia, it is most undesirable to damage this nerve by pricking it accidentally.

6.3.3　Technical aspects

Only a single injection is required to anaesthetise the mandibular nerve, i.e. the inferior alveolar and lingual nerve. An aspirating cartridge syringe is used with a 25-gauge needle that is 35 mm long. When anaesthetising the mandibular nerve, the point of the needle is placed in the pterygomandibular space. This space is bordered ventrally by the mucosa of the pharyngeal arches. This is where the injection needle is inserted in the pterygomandibular space. This space is bordered laterally by the ascending branch of the lower jaw and dorsally by the median part of the parotid gland and the skin. The attachment of the medial pterygoid muscle is found caudally and also borders the space median. The lateral pterygoid muscle borders the space cranially.

The mandibular nerve, inferior alveolar nerve, lingual nerve, buccal nerve and branches of the arteries and maxillary veins run within the space. The space runs ventro-caudally into the submandibular space and caudo-cranially into the parapharyngeal and retropharyngeal spaces, which eventually lead to the mediastinum and pericardium.

6.4   The direct and indirect technique

The inside of the mandibular ramus is more or less divergent dorsally. Therefore, various techniques can be used to anaesthetise the mandibular nerve ('mandibular block'). A distinction must be made between the so-called direct and indirect technique. The direct technique is performed from the homolateral side. The risk of this is that the anaesthetic fluid may be applied too far medially. This has led to the indirect technique, which is performed from the contralateral commissure. The danger of this is that the medial pterygoid muscle may be damaged or anaesthetic fluid may be injected into this muscle. This would lead to postoperative trismus, which may persist for days or weeks, or to a haematoma. The direct technique does not have these risks, but lacks the relative certainty of a truly effective anaesthesia.

For administration of anaesthesia with either the direct or the indirect technique, a number of characteristic anatomical structures are of great importance. The following anatomical structures determine the place, direction and penetration depth of the needle:

- *The plane of occlusion.* Anaesthesia is given parallel to the plane of occlusion, approx. one finger width above (1–1.5 cm).
- *The deepest point of the front of the mandibular ramus.* If the non-injecting hand feels along the front of the ramus, the entrance of the mandibular canal appears to be on the same level as the deepest point.
- *The triangle at the front of the pterygomandibular space* that is formed by the cheek mucosa that runs into the throat and pterygomandibular plica running from the palate to the retromolar pad. The needle must be inserted in the middle of this triangle.
- The thumb of the non-injecting hand feels along the front of the ramus, while three fingers of the same hand feel along the back of the ramus. Exactly halfway between the thumb and fingers is the *mandibular foramen*, where the alveolar nerve enters the jaw. In adults the foramen is found exactly in between the front and back. In children the foramen lies about a third in from the front. This determines the depth of the needle's insertion (Figure 6.7).

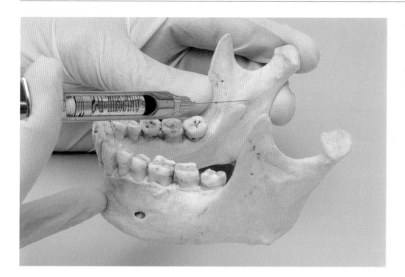

Figure 6.7
Lingual aspect of an adult mandibula with the lingula exactly in the middle between the front and back sides.

With the *indirect* technique the anaesthesia is given from the contralateral commissure and the syringe is moved to the middle of the mouth opening while the needle is pushed in. With the *direct technique* the anaesthesia is given from the homolateral corner of the mouth and the syringe is moved to the middle of the mouth opening if necessary while the needle is inserted. Whilst inserting the needle, the dentist must attempt to move the needle as close to the bone as possible without touching the periosteum unnecessarily. It is also important to hold the tip of the needle in such a way that it does not get stuck in the periosteum.

The thumb of the non-injecting hand seeks for the deepest point of the right ramus and the fingers feel along the back of it. The needle is held parallel to the plane of occlusion, about one finger width above it. The needle point is then inserted in the middle of the mucosa triangle until it makes contact with the bone. Following this, the needle is carefully pushed up by moving the syringe to the middle of the oral cavity and holding it parallel to the plane of occlusion. The level of divergence inside the mandibular ramus differs from person to person. When 1 cm of the needle still remains visible and the point is exactly in the middle between the front and back of the ramus, the dentist carefully aspirates. Approximately 1.5 ml of anaesthetic fluid is injected (Figure 6.8). The needle is then pulled back about 1 cm and the dentist aspirates once again. The rest of the carpule is then injected in order to anaesthetise the lingual nerve (Figure 6.9).

Now the syringe is taken out of the mouth. The patient closes the mouth and is given a compliment for his/her cooperation during the anaesthesia. The dentist also asks about the patient's experience: 'Was it painful? Do you feel the effects of the anaesthesia?' If necessary, the cartridge is replaced and anaesthesia is given to the buccal nerve, also one finger-width above the point of occlusion exactly on the front side of the ramus. Here the buccal nerve, running from high lingual, crosses the front side on its way

Figure 6.8 A
Mandibular block
anaesthesia. The drawing
shows the position of the
needle point in relation to the
mandibular foramen.

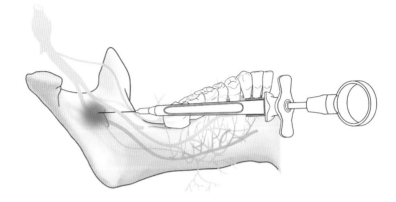

Figure 6.8 B1 and B2
The technique of mandibular
block anaesthesia from the
left corner of the mouth
(indirect technique). The
needle is inserted to the bone,
pulled back a millimetre and
then the syringe is moved to
the middle of the mouth and
carefully pushed in so that
about 1 cm of the needle
remains visible. The injection
is given after aspiration.

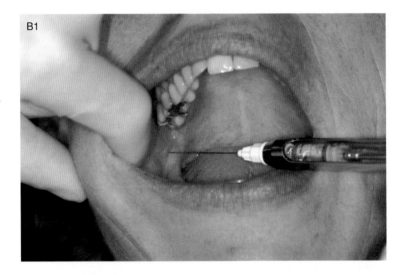

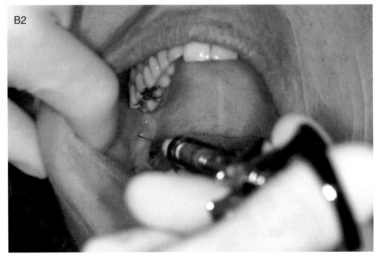

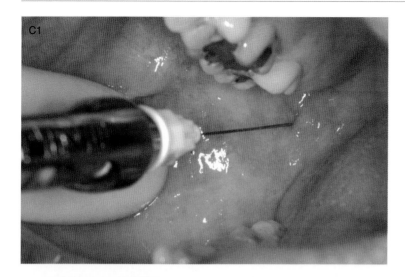

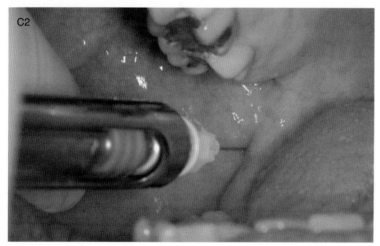

Figure 6.8 C1 and C2
Mandibular block anaesthesia
from the right corner of the
mouth (direct technique).
The mouth is opened as much
as possible and the needle is
inserted carefully on the
lingual side of the mandibular
ramus so that 1 cm of the
needle remains visible.
The injection is given
after aspiration.

down to the gingiva and mucosa in the region M_3–P_{1inf} (Figure 6.10). The path of the buccal nerve varies, however, so that the dentist may elect to give an infiltration anaesthesia buccal to the element to be anaesthetised.

About 2–3 minutes after giving a mandibular block the patient should indicate that the corner of the mouth, lower lip, edge and tip of the tongue have begun to tingle and feel odd. One minute later the lower lip and tongue will be anaesthetised on one side and the treatment can start.

An experienced dentist, who takes the characteristic anatomical structures that were previously mentioned into account, will achieve a good mandibular anaesthesia in about 85% of cases. Block anaesthesia may fail due to individual anatomical differences, such as a progenic mandibula, a divergent angle between the horizontal and vertical part of the mandibula, or the absence of teeth.

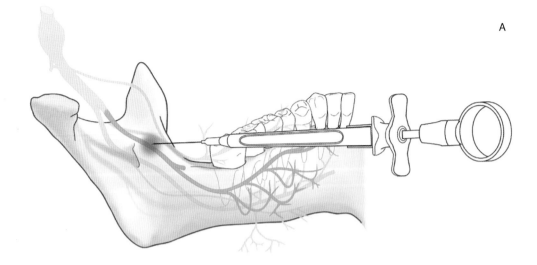

A

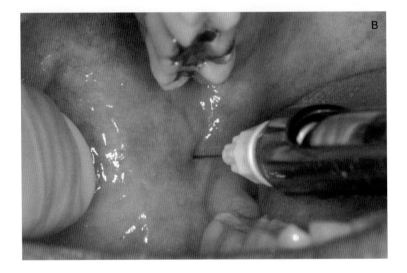

B

Figure 6.9 A and B
Drawing (**A**) and photo (**B**) of block anaesthesia of the lingual nerve right. After a mandibular block the needle is pulled back about 1 cm. The injection is given after aspiration.

Failing of the lingula is the most common reason for an ineffective mandibular block. The point of the injection needle is then found to be too far medially, too low or too far dorsally. Other complications may also occur. In approximately 15% of cases, blood is aspirated. It is also possible for the needle to touch the lingual nerve or the inferior alveolar nerve. In the case of positive aspiration or when a nerve has been touched, it is enough to pull the needle back a few millimetres. If the needle is in too deep, this can lead to local anaesthesia within the capsule of the parotid gland. This may result in one-sided paralysis of the facial nerve, which fortunately lasts only a few hours.

When the mandibular block is not effective, another injection may be given. There is a chance that, during the second injection, the patient will

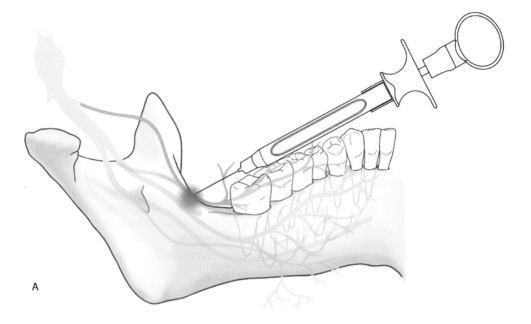

A

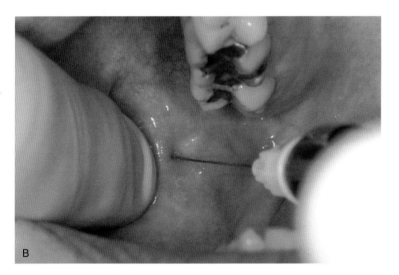

B

not notice a touching of the lingual nerve, the inferior alveolar nerve or the mandibular nerve by the needle. The nerve may then be damaged without the patient or dentist noticing. It is therefore advisable to employ intraligamentous anaesthesia, particularly if the lingual nerve and the inferior alveolar nerve are not anaesthetised. An additional injection also has the disadvantage that an 'acidic environment' slowly develops inside the pterygomandibular space due to the addition of another 1.7–1.8 ml of anaesthetic fluid with a low pH. In this environment, the ionised form of anaesthetic will increase. This form is unable to pass through the myelin sheath, thus reducing the effectiveness of the local anaesthetic.

Figure 6.10 A and B
Drawing (**A**) and photo (**B**) of block anaesthesia of the buccal nerve that runs from high lingual, crosses the front of the ramus (at the level of the finger) and then runs down to low buccal.

Mandibular anaesthesia on the left side of the patient is conducted in the same way as on the right side. The only difference is that the left hand injects instead of the right hand. If a dentist still prefers to use the right hand, he/she must move to an 11–12 o'clock position. The left hand holds the patient's cheek to the side and feels along the front of the mandibular ramus, while the right hand gives the anaesthetic.

In some situations, such as two-sided extractions in the lower jaw, extensive periodontal treatment and (pre-)implantological treatments in the interforaminal area, a two-sided mandibular block may be given to healthy patients. The entire mandibula is then anaesthetised, including the lower lip and the front two-thirds of the tongue. The tongue's motorics remain undisturbed, however, as well as reflexive swallowing. Reflexive swallowing begins at the back third of the tongue and pharynx. Because the foremost part of the tongue is anaesthetised, the patient will not notice if anything is lying on it, such as a broken part of a molar or a piece of filling. The dentist and assistant must, therefore, keep a good eye on the oral cavity and throat.

6.5 Molars

6.5.1 Anatomical aspects

Both on the buccal and on the lingual side, the roots of the molars are covered by a thick layer of cortical bone. The external oblique rim and the mylohyoid rim form an extra barrier for the diffusion of anaesthetic fluid to the apices of the molars (Figure 6.11). The roots of the molars lie on the lingual side, usually below the level of the mylohyoid muscle and buccal to the M_{2inf} under the point of attachment of the buccinator muscle. Infiltration of these muscles must be avoided as a haematoma increases the risk of infection.

Figure 6.11

Anatomical drawing of the inferior alveolar nerve and its branches to the apices of the molars.

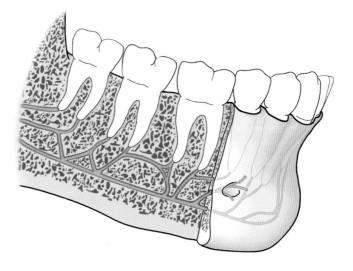

6.5.2 Indication

Cavity preparations, endodontic treatment and surgical treatments require a mandibular block, supplemented by block or infiltration anaesthesia of the buccal nerve. Intraligamentous anaesthesia should, theoretically, also suffice for cavity preparations and endodontic treatments.

6.5.3 Technique

See the text above for the technical aspects of a mandibular block and buccal nerve anaesthesia.

6.6 Third molars in the lower jaw

6.6.1 Anatomical aspects

The impacted M_{3inf} lies in the mandibular angle region, dorsal to the M_{2inf}. This area is innervated not only by the mandibular nerve but also by sensory branches that leave the spinal column at C2 and C3, and run over the platysma to the angle. This must be taken into account when surgically removing the M_{3inf}.

The lingual nerve runs caudo-laterally from its source in the direction of the jaw and is found at the height of the M_{3inf} approx. 5 mm lingually and caudally to the bone edge, and dorsally to the M_{2inf}. The path of the lingual nerve, however, shows great individual variation: the lingual nerve can also be found on the lingual side of the alveolar process above the impacted M_{3inf} at the height of the bone (Figure 6.12).

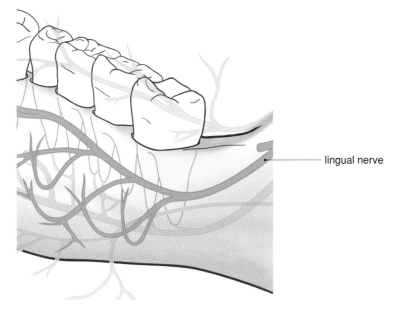

lingual nerve

Figure 6.12
Lingual aspect of the mandibula with the M_{3inf} and lingual nerve relation right.

6.6.2   Indication

Surgical treatments such as trigone bone transplant, an operculectomy
and removal of the (partly) impacted M_{3inf} require mandibular block
anaesthesia and anaesthesia of the buccal nerve. If the M_{3inf} is deeply
impacted, anaesthesia is also needed for the sensory branches from C2
and C3 by applying infiltration anaesthesia deep in the fold behind the
M_{2inf}.

6.6.3   Technique

See the text above for the mandibular block technique and block
anaesthesia of the buccal nerve.

7 Additional anaesthetic techniques

J.A. Baart

In dentistry, infiltration anaesthesia of the maxillary nerve (Chapter 5) is mainly used for anaesthetising the teeth and surrounding tissues of the upper jaw. In the lower jaw, block anaesthesia of the mandibular nerve (Chapter 6) is usually applied. In this chapter, several supplementary anaesthetic techniques are discussed, such as regional block anaesthesia of the maxillary, infraorbital, nasopalatine and mental nerves. The Gow-Gates technique, an alternative to mandibular block anaesthesia, is also described.

7.1 Maxillary nerve block

Blockade of the maxillary nerve induces anaesthesia of half of the maxilla, which enables surgical treatment in the upper jaw and maxillary sinus under local anaesthesia. This regional block can also be used to counteract pain in cases of inexplicable pain complaints. A maxillary nerve block can be achieved via high tuberosity anaesthesia or via the greater palatine foramen. A local anaesthetic with vasoconstrictor is used, applied with an aspirating syringe and a 25-gauge needle (bent at approximately 45 degrees).

7.1.1 High tuberosity anaesthesia

The maxillary nerve leaves the skull through the foramen rotundum. The nerve runs through the pterygopalatine fossa and then on through the orbit as the infraorbital nerve. The infraorbital nerve runs through a canal at the bottom of the orbit and leaves the canal again through the infraorbital foramen.

The pterygopalatine fossa is accessible from the mouth. This fossa can be reached with a 35-mm-long 25-gauge needle if the needle is bent to approximately 45 degrees. This bent needle must pass the mucosa behind the zygomaticoalveolar crest, about 1 cm from the alveolar process, and then be directed dorso-medially (Figure 7.1). After aspiration, about one cartridge may be injected. Two to three minutes later, half of the upper jaw will be anaesthetised. In some cases the infraorbital nerve is insufficiently numbed by this technique. Furthermore, there is a chance of injecting into

Figure 7.1 A and B

Photos of skull (**A**) and patient (**B**) show a high tuberosity anaesthesia. The (bent) needle is inserted from out to in, high in the pterygopalatine fossa, just by the split of the maxillary nerve into the infraorbital and superior alveolar nerves. The injection is given after aspiration.

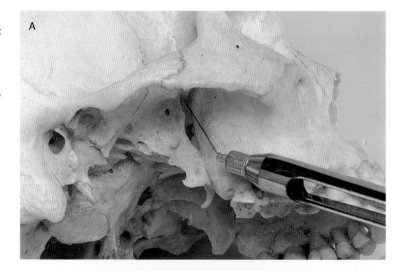

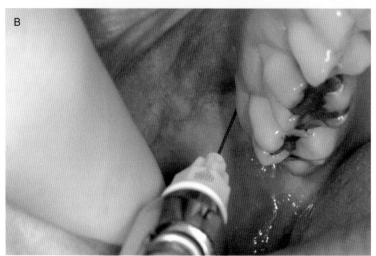

the pterygoid plexus, so that there is a risk of intravasal injection and developing a haematoma.

7.1.2   Greater palatine foramen block

A greater palatine foramen block is used less frequently than high tuberosity anaesthesia, but can be easily carried out intraorally. The greater palatine foramen lies approximately 1 cm palatinally to the M_2–M_3 region and approximately 0.5 cm in front of the pterygoid hamulus. The direction of the canal is 45 degrees to dorsal in relation to the occlusion plane. The bent needle is carefully inserted into the foramen, and by inserting the needle slowly, the entire length of the needle can be used (Figure 7.2). After aspiration, a half to one cartridge may be injected. Within 2–3 minutes, half of the maxilla will be anaesthetised.

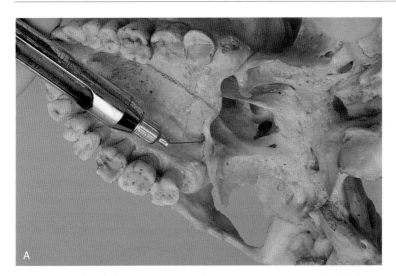

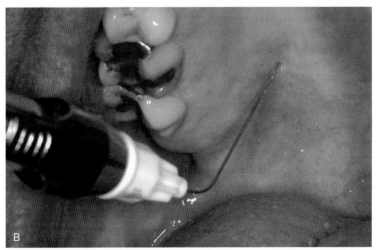

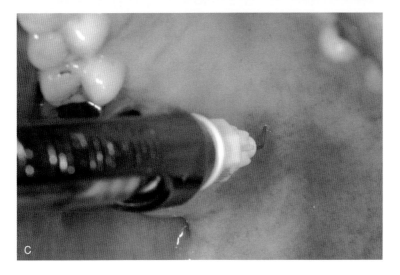

Figure 7.2 A, B and C
Photo of skull (**A**) and photos of patient (**B** and **C**) show a maxillary nerve block via the greater palatine foramen. The needle is bent approx. 45 degrees and inserted in the foramen, which is located approx. 1 cm palatinal to the M_2–M_3 region. The cartridge syringe is held parallel to the occlusion plain of the upper jaw. The needle can now be pushed in carefully. The injection is performed after aspiration.

It is not always easy to find the entrance to the foramen. Moreover, inserting the needle roughly can lead to long-term damage of the nerve. Finally, if the patient has a small maxilla, the anaesthetic fluid may reach the parasympathetic sphenopalatine ganglion so that unintended side effects may occur, such as diplopia (double vision).

7.2   Infraorbital nerve block

The infraorbital nerve runs almost horizontally through the canal in the orbital floor until it leaves through the infraorbital foramen, approximately 5–10 mm caudally to the infraorbital rim. The nerve supplies sensibility to the nostril, cheek, lower eyelid, upper lip, gingiva and upper frontal teeth.

An infraorbital nerve block is suitable for the dental treatment and surgery of frontal teeth. A vasoconstrictor containing anaesthetic is used for this block, applied with a customary cartridge syringe with a 25-gauge needle of 25–35 mm. There are two intraoral methods for blocking the infraorbital nerve. The first involves the needle being positioned approximately 0.5 cm laterally from P_{2sup}, whilst the other method involves the needle being inserted approximately 1 cm from the alveolar process of C_{sup}. The lip is lifted with the thumb, and the index finger of the same hand feels the infraorbital rim extraorally. The needle is then moved in the direction of the finger. With the method in which the needle is inserted in the buccal sulcus at the level of the C_{sup}, the needle is directed towards the pupil of the eye (Figure 7.3). With the 'P_{2sup} method', the needle is inserted in the direction of the longitudinal axis of this tooth. After about 2 cm the needle will make contact with the bone at the level of the infraorbital foramen. The unaltered position of the index finger prevents the needle from being fed in so far that it touches the eyelid or eyeball. A depot of half a cartridge is enough.

The method is simple, effective and safe. However, if a vein or small artery is damaged, a haematoma may occur directly under the eyelid, and touching the nerve with the needle leads to prolonged anaesthesia and paraesthesia.

7.3   Nasopalatine nerve block

The nasopalatine nerve, which runs over the floor of the nose through the incisor canal to the incisive papilla, provides sensibility to the anterior third of the palate. Anaesthesia of this nerve is appropriate for crown preparations in the entire upper front and for surgical treatment, such as ligating or removing an impacted canine, periodontal surgery and implantology.

An anaesthetic with a vasoconstrictor is administered with a regular cartridge syringe with a 25-gauge needle at least 20 mm long. With the mouth open, the needle point is placed right on the incisive papilla. The needle is introduced slowly, parallel to the direction of the buccal cortical

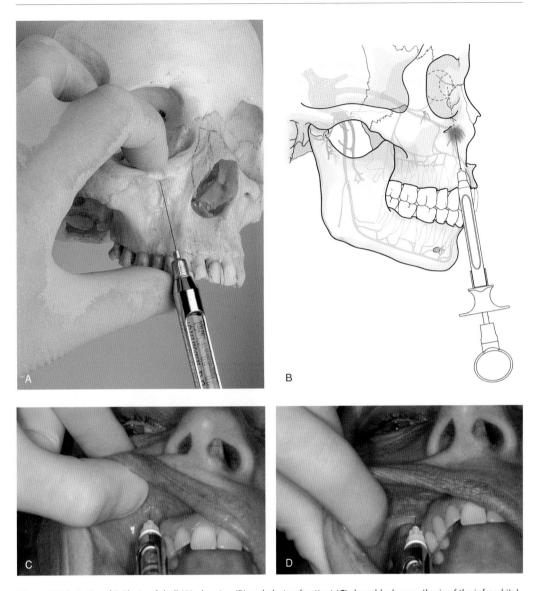

Figure 7.3 A, B, C and D Photo of skull (**A**), drawing (**B**) and photo of patient (**C**) show block anaesthesia of the infraorbital nerve. The needle is inserted 1 cm vestibular to the C_{sup} right and is inserted in the direction of the pupil. The index finger of the non-injecting hand rests on the infraorbital rim. The injection is given after aspiration. Photo of patient (**D**) shows an alternative method, where the needle is inserted straight up from the buccal sulcus of the P_1–P_{2sup} right region so that it stops at the level of the infraorbital foramen.

bone contour (Figure 7.4). This is almost vertical in some patients; for others it is inclined dorsally. The direction is important to avoid the needle getting stuck in the canal or having to be reinserted because it can no longer follow the canal. After approximately 1 cm a quarter cartridge is injected very slowly.

Figure 7.4 A and B

Photo of skull (**A**) and photo of patient (**B**) show block anaesthesia of the nasopalatine nerve. The needle is inserted upright into the incisive papilla and introduced carefully for approx. 1 cm into the nasopalatine canal. This runs parallel to the axis direction of the central incisor. The injection is given after aspiration.

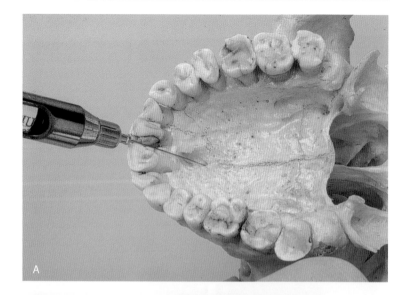

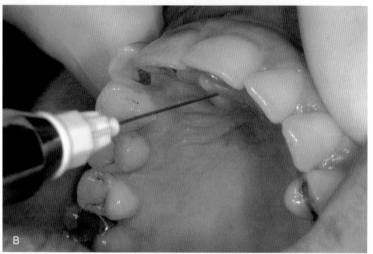

This injection technique is painful, even in expert hands. With explanation, precision and expertise, however, this anaesthesia can be used very successfully with children, e.g. for ligating an impacted canine or removing a mesiodens. If the nerve is damaged, an anaesthetised area may arise at the anterior of the palate durum and last for 3–4 months.

7.4   Mental nerve block

The mental nerve leaves the mandibular canal via the mental foramen approximately 5–8 mm under the P_1–P_{2inf} apices and provides sensitivity to

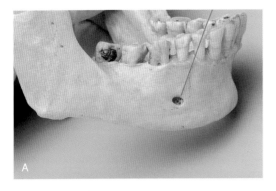

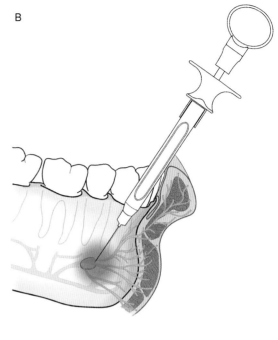

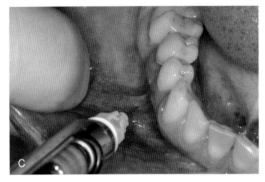

the lower lip, skin of the chin and oral mucosa, ventral to the foramen. The lower frontal teeth, including P_{1inf}, are not innervated by the mental nerve.

Blocking the mental nerve is advised for surgery of the lower lip and the anterior edentous alveolar process front, and for biopsy of the relevant area. A cartridge syringe with a short 25-gauge needle is used, and a local anaesthetic with vasoconstrictor. The mouth is almost closed and the thumb holds the lip to the side. The fingers of the same hand feel the inferior border of the mandible. The short needle penetrates the mucosa by the P_{1inf}, approximately 0.5 cm from the alveolar process. The needle point is introduced slightly medially and dorsally, so that contact with the bone occurs after approximately 1.5 cm (Figure 7.5). Half a cartridge is injected after aspiration. The half lower lip, skin of the chin and buccal mucosa are anaesthetised within 2–3 minutes.

If the needle is inserted too far dorsally, the foramen will be missed. When the needle is inserted too far laterally, the fluid will accumulate subcutaneously.

Additional infiltration anaesthesia is often needed for surgery of the soft parts of the lip area, because of the vasconstrictive effect. A small injection is sufficient at the level of the corner of the mouth, where the labial artery reaches the lip area.

Figure 7.5 A, B and C
Photo of skull (**A**), drawing (**B**) and photo of patient (**C**) show block anaesthesia of the mental nerve, for anaesthetising half of the lower lip/chin area right, including the buccal mucosa. The needle is introduced approx. 1.5 cm. An injection is given after aspiration.

7.5   Gow-Gates technique

Usually the direct or indirect technique is selected for a mandibular block (see Section 6.4), where two consecutive injections anaesthetise first the inferior alveolar nerve and lingual nerve and second the buccal nerve. In 1973, the Australian George Gow-Gates described a block anaesthesia that is a mandibular block at a much higher level. This method anaesthetises the entire mandibular nerve with a single depot, so that an additional block of the lingual or buccal nerve is no longer necessary.

The chance of a successful anaesthesia of the entire mandibular nerve following the Gow-Gates technique is about 95%. The success rate of a classical inferior alveolar nerve block is 85%. The advantages of the Gow-Gates technique, however, are limited.

The thumb feels along the attachment of the temporal muscles to the coronoid process. Medial to this, the needle is inserted into the mucosa at the height of the occlusal plane of the M_{2sup}. The index finger of the same hand is placed in the external auditory canal and the needle is then inserted about 25–27 mm in the direction of the index finger. Bone contact is made with the medioventral side of the condyle (Figure 7.6).

It is necessary to aspirate because the needle point may enter the maxillary artery. After aspiration, an entire cartridge of anaesthetic fluid is injected. After 2–3 minutes the following branches of the mandibular nerve will be anaesthetised: the inferior alveolar nerve, the lingual nerve and almost always the buccal nerve. If the needle is introduced too far, the mandibular caput may be missed and the needle will shift over the mandibular incisura into the masseteric muscle.

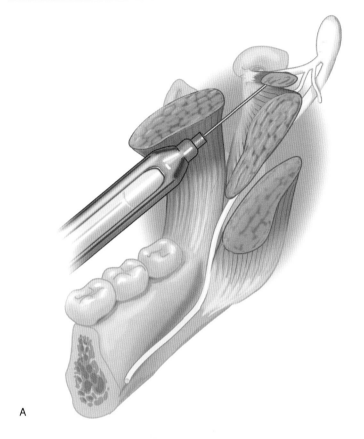

Figure 7.6 A and B
Drawing (**A**) and photo of patient (**B**) show the Gow-Gates technique for anaesthesia of the mandibular nerve. On the lingual side of the coronoid process, at the height of the M_{2sup} the needle is inserted in the mucosa in the direction of the external auditory canal. The needle is introduced almost completely until bone contact is made with the medioventral side of the condyle.

A

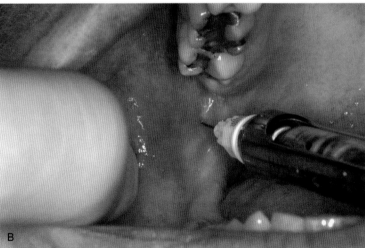

B

8 Local anaesthesia for children

F.W.A. Frankenmolen

Needless to say, children tend to dread local anaesthesia. The dentist may deal with this in various ways. He/she must win the trust of the child, speak in a manner the child understands, use an injection technique that is effective and does not cause the child any pain, and know and prevent complications. Finally, the dentist must treat the child with empathy.

8.1 Introduction

Dental treatment may sometimes be unpleasant for children. They may find it threatening, they may be afraid of possible pain, and the specific dental sounds and smells may arouse feelings of discomfort. As a consequence, some children are already afraid of the dentist at a very young age. A good relationship of trust between child and dentist as well as painless treatment are essential for child-friendly and adequate dental care.

The dental team must be aware of factors that the child may experience as uncomfortable, and that may be stored in the child's memory. The manner in which children experience events, the way parents view the treatment of their child, and also the way in which the dentist and dental assistant deal with the child's behaviour are important factors contributing to a child's positive memory of dental treatment.

If children go to the dentist regularly, their fear will, in most cases, not increase. Regular visits to the dentist can help to prevent an aggravating treatment having long-term effects. Psychological research has shown that some children are more sensitive than others to what happens to them and are therefore more vulnerable to various interventional situations. They develop fear of the dentist faster than other children. Therefore, vulnerable children must always be treated painlessly and in the same way. This requires a very consistent method of treatment, so that children always know in advance what to expect. In order to prevent painful treatment, it is advisable to anaesthetise children. Moreover, an anaesthetic can prevent undesirable behaviour during the treatment from escalating unnecessarily.

8.2 Experience of pain and fear in children

Not all children react in the same way to (supposed) pain impulses, and pain thresholds seem to vary greatly between children. A toddler may fall down the stairs and, though bruised, may be quickly comforted by the mother or father with a kiss where it hurts. The same toddler may cry inconsolably while fissures on a tooth are being sealed, because the child may expect it to hurt (Box 8.1).

Box 8.1

Sander (aged 4): "I don't want any needle"
For small children, fear of anaesthesia is very difficult to analyse into parts. They are very quickly afraid of the whole situation because a part of it is threatening. On the other hand, they are easy to reassure and are responsive to help and support. The dentist achieves much by simply explaining everything calmly, taking the initiative and proceeding with the treatment. Attempting dental treatment without anaesthesia will usually only increase the stress, so that in many cases further treatment is no longer possible at all.

Anna (aged 9): "Must it really be with anaesthesia?"
When children are older they start to think, to anticipate and sometimes also to worry more. The dentist must then respond according to the level of fear. An explanation should be given, the necessity of the treatment must be explained clearly, and alternatives discussed, as appropriate: start without anaesthesia; then if that does not work, give an anaesthetic. The rational value of this approach increases the child's confidence in the reliability of the dentist.

Mandy (aged 3) is the boss at home and now also in the dental office. She knows that her parents will get out of bed at night if she cries hard and long enough. As a reward she gets something nice to drink and that has led to obvious damage to her teeth. As the dentist explains that her teeth are going to sleep and will wake up better and prettier, her "I don't want it" attitude takes over, emphasised by her attempts to make a dramatic get-away. The dentist is too quick for her, however, but she does not give up. Mandy then applies her proven method and starts to scream, which can be heard way beyond the waiting room. The dentist responds and promises to try again next time, thereby signing his own death warrant.

John (aged 4) has "mustles"
John can hardly be convinced of the necessity of local anaesthesia. Instead his mother says with a smile, "You know, John, you have to sleep well to get strong muscles. Now your tooth has to sleep to get strong for cleaning and a small filling." He agrees to that. He nods and lies back with his arms crossed. Now giving the anaesthetic is easy. When the needle is barely out of his mouth, he sits up and shows his arms: "Mum, have I got mustles now?"

During a child's life, he or she may be afraid of a series of events. Most fears subside, because the child learns to understand the situation and learns to cope with it. Coping with fears differs from child to child and coping mechanisms change with age. The most universal coping mechanism is to avoid a scary situation. Unfortunately, avoidance behaviour is also a coping style that fully confirms the fear (Box 8.2).

Box 8.2

A child requires an approach that corresponds to his or her age, an approach that offers security and support in a sometimes new and therefore 'insecure' situation. Sitting in the dental chair, each child is especially interested in his or her own safety. The child does not really know what the dentist is about to do and, if he/she does know, the child may often dread the treatment and will not – or hardly – be able to deal with it.

Young children can find support in fearful situations from a parent's hug. However, they may also express their fear by crying a lot or by trying to run away. As children grow older, they are better able to deal with scary situations. They may fantasise and/or resist verbally. The older they get, the more they understand, so that situations that first made them afraid appear far less scary. In more uncomfortable cases, older children may choose from several strategies, for example discussion or negotiation. However, they also have the choice of direct actions, such as learning to relax if they have a fear of needles or knowing what they can do or think about in order to calm down.

A remarkable aspect of coping in young children is that they do not regard themselves as afraid. One should not be surprised if a young child, who has been crying a lot during dental treatment, afterwards tells his mother quite contentedly that it went well, it did not hurt and he had not cried(!). The crying during the dental treatment was a coping mechanism for keeping control in an uncomfortable situation, and much less a sign that the dentist was doing anything wrong.

When children get older, they can distinguish very well between fear and coping. It is harder to tell from their behaviour, but when asked they can express clearly what they are afraid of and how they deal with it. They know exactly in which situations they need support, when they just need to concentrate and what they fear so much they are unable to deal with.

8.2.1 Security and support

Young children look for security in new or alien situations (Figure 8.1). If they are restless, tense or nervous, the presence of a familiar person will calm them and give support. If parents or carers have had a mixture of positive and negative experiences, they often have a more balanced

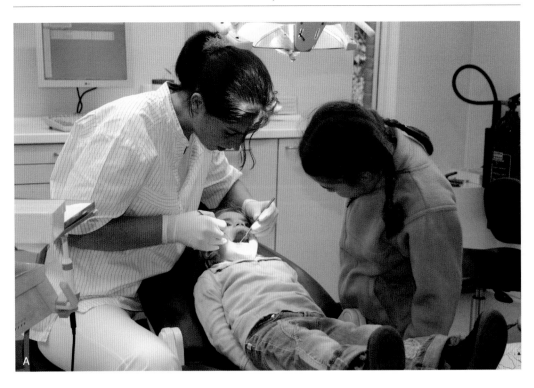

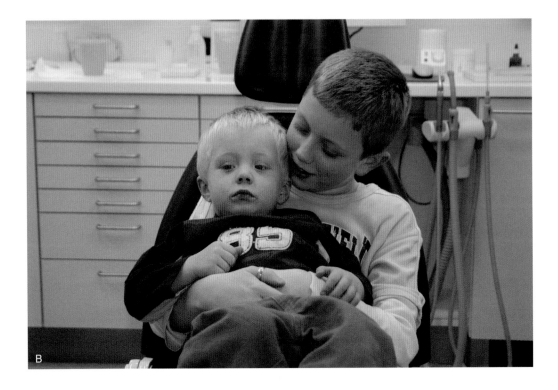

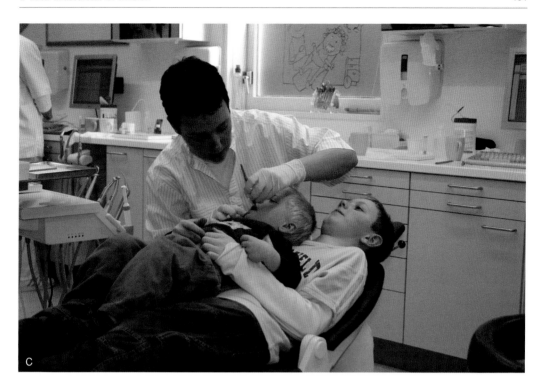

attitude. The more negative cases parents have experienced, the more they will be on alert and the sooner they want to warn and protect their child. This is the general case and is also the case for the dentist, especially when using anaesthesia.

If the parent him/herself is scared, the child's reaction will be the signal to express very negative emotions that the parent has from his/her own dental history. The parent may rush to the child to protect him or her, saying reassuringly, "The dentist isn't scary at all" or "The injection really won't hurt". With this, parents will bring out an aspect that only evokes more fear in the child. Essentially, what they are saying is: "Watch out, there is danger!" and strengthen that signal with attention: "Come now, you're safe with me".

Parents can be a support to the child during dental treatment (Box 8.3). However, if a scared parent accompanies the child, this may mean that the child chooses a coping strategy that does not work with the dental treatment being performed. In order to deal with this situation effectively, the dentist must explain this phenomenon to the parent and perform the treatment without the presence of the parent, either at that session or at the next appointment. It is important that the parent understands he/she is not being punished for his/her behaviour, but that the relationship between the child and dentist will be improved if the parent is not present.

Figure 8.1 A, B and C
Security and support.

Box 8.3

It goes without saying that a good relationship with the child's parent or carer is of great importance and time must be set aside for a thorough explanation of the treatment. In such a situation, the parent or carer can more easily give suggestions for the way the dental team could best approach his or her child. A positive attitude of the parent or carer is a good starting point for a favourable approach of the child.

8.2.2   Preparation for anaesthesia

If the dentist assumes that the treatment will cause pain, it is important to prepare the child, and also the parent or carer, timely for the administration of local anaesthesia. It is important that the parent or carer also receives concrete information about how the child can be prepared for the treatment with regard to behaviour and practically. For the child, a simple explanation is important. The parent or carer can be shown with models or X-rays that there is a real chance of pain in certain situations and that this pain may be prevented with local anaesthesia.

An important aspect is the health of the child. Most dentists assume that children are healthy. Research shows, however, that approximately 10% of children between the ages of 0 and 18 have health problems. It is clear that during the intake of a young patient, but also prior to anaesthetising children, a medical history should be taken. Figure 8.2 provides an example of a medical questionnaire for children.

8.2.3   Child-friendly procedure

As already mentioned, the child must receive information about the 'how' and 'wherefore' of the local anaesthetic. Almost all children will nod in agreement if the dentist tells them, "I think your tooth wants to have a nice sleep while we clean it".

Value-laden words such as 'injection', 'anaesthetic', 'needle' and 'syringe' are better replaced by terms like 'putting the tooth to sleep' and 'sleepy juice'. In fact, any description is fine as long as it is used consistently. In the same way, the use of the phrase 'to notice' instead of 'to feel' can avoid undesirable reactions, since 'to notice' is a more neutral term than 'to feel.'

It does no harm to show the child the syringe prior to the injection, but it is not necessary (Figure 8.3). If the dentist feels doubtful about this, it is not necessary to show the cartridge syringe during the explanation.

While explaining the procedure, it is advisable to mention the bitter taste of the anaesthetic ointment and/or anaesthetic fluid. It is a pity if the anaesthetic is administered faultlessly, but the child panics from the horrid taste of the anaesthetic fluid. When the dentist demonstrates the syringe,

Instruction to complete this form

If you have answered the main question with **NO**, you may skip the sub-questions

Date   :
Name   :
Date of birth   :
Address   :
Telephone number :
Name of general physician :

Permission to exchange information with general physician
Signature parent/carer:

Medical risk from the anamnesis

....
....

1. **Is your child under treatment (currently or previously) by a (general) physician, psychologist or medical specialist?**   **YES**   **NO**
    If yes,
    At which hospital? ....
    In which department? ....
    Under which physician?...
    For what?...
2. **Does your child have lung or respiratory diseases (COPD, asthma, bronchitis, frequent cough, pneumonia)?**   **YES**   **NO**
    If yes,
    Is your child currently suffering from this?   yes   no
    Is medication working insufficiently?   yes   no
    Does your child suffer from shortness of breath?   yes   no
3. **Does your child have a heart murmur or a congenital heart defect?**   **YES**   **NO**
    If yes,
    Has your child ever had acute rheumatic fever?   **YES**   **NO**
    If yes,
    Are antibiotics necessary for dental treatment?   yes   no
    Are there symptoms of the cardiac disease?   yes   no
4. **Did your child have cardiac surgery?**   **YES**   **NO**
    If yes,
    For what?..
    Did your child have an artificial heart valve fitted?   yes   no
    Have symptoms remained after treatment?   yes   no
5. **Does your child have heart rhythm problems?**   **YES**   **NO**
    If yes,
    Must your child avoid physical activities?   yes   no
    Must your child sit or lay down during attacks?   yes   no
6. **Does your child have epilepsy?**   **YES**   **NO**
    If yes,
    Is the medication changed frequently?   yes   no
    Does you child have frequent attacks, despite the medication?   yes   no
7. **Does your child have diabetes?**   **YES**   **NO**
    If yes,
    Is your child treated with insulin?   yes   no
    Is your child frequently disregulated?   yes   no
8. **Does your child have anaemia?**   **YES**   **NO**
    If yes,
    Is your child frequently tired or dizzy?   yes   no
    Is there a family member with congenital anaemia?   yes   no
9. **Does your child have a bleeding tendency?**   **YES**   **NO**
    If yes,
    Do wounds heal slowly or keep bleeding for a long time?   yes   no
    Does your child spontaneously bruise or get a bleeding nose?   yes   no
    Is there a family member with a bleeding tendency?   yes   no
10. **Does your child currently have a contagious disease?**   **YES**   **NO**
    If yes,
    Which? ....

Figure 8.2
Medical questionnaire for children (Academic Centre for Dentistry Amsterdam, ACTA).

Figure 8.2

Cont'd

11. Has your child had any childhood diseases?	**YES**	**NO**
If yes,		
Which?		
Does (or did) your child suffer from frequent infections		
e.g. inflammation of the ear?	**YES**	**NO**
Which?		
12. Does your child currently have a liver disease?	**YES**	**NO**
If yes,		
Has he/she been hospitalised for this?	yes	no
Is your child using medication or a diet?	yes	no
Is your child a carrier of a hepatitis virus?	yes	no
13. Is your child allergic?	**YES**	**NO**
If yes,		
Pollen or grass (hay fever)	yes	no
Rubber/latex	yes	no
Iodine	yes	no
Plasters	yes	no
Soy	yes	no
Gluten	yes	no
Anaesthesia	yes	no
Antibiotics (penicillin)	yes	no
Other		
Does your child use medication for the allergy?	**YES**	**NO**
If yes,		
Which?		
14. Did your child ever have unexpected reactions during or		
after dental treatment?	**YES**	**NO**
If yes,		
What were the complications?		
Which dentist gave the treatment?		
15. Is your child prescribed medication (e.g. by a general		
physician or medical specialist)?	**YES**	**NO**
If yes,		
Aspirin or other painkillers	yes	no
For asthma	yes	no
Tranquillisers	yes	no
Prednisone, corticosteroids or other immunosuppressive drugs	yes	no
Medication against cancer or blood diseases	yes	no
Penicillin or other antibiotics	yes	no
For diabetes	yes	no
For epilepsy	yes	no
Other		
16. Does your child suffer from any disease or condition that		
has not been covered above?	**YES**	**NO**
If yes,		
Which?		

droplets could be dripped onto the child's finger, for example, so he/she knows how bitter it tastes. This clarifies to the child why it is good to suction saliva so that the bitter taste does not spread through the mouth. The pressure of the suction tube on the mucosa can serve as an extra distraction from the insertion of the needle.

8.2.4   Warning

The numbness and stiffness of the soft tissue, which persist long after the dental treatment, are unavoidable but sometimes also dangerous side effects of local anaesthesia in children. Only the administration of local anaesthesia through the periodontal ligament avoids these problems.

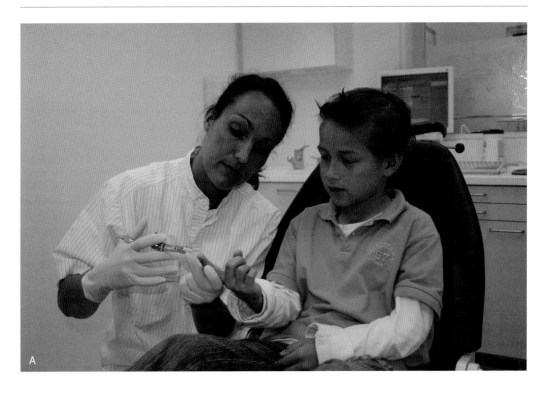

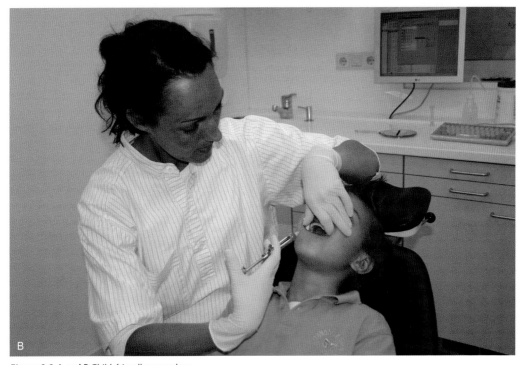

Figure 8.3 A and B Child-friendly procedure.

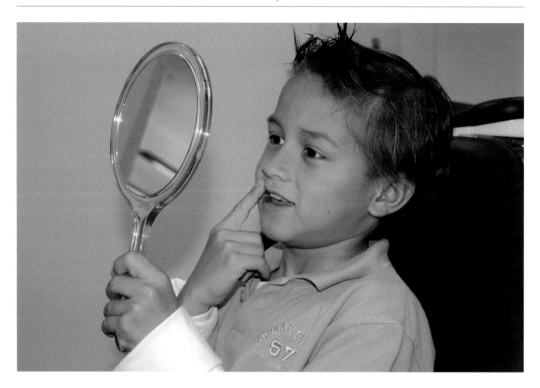

Figure 8.4
Children can express the numbness with the use of a mirror. The lip feels swollen but is not.

Children can express their experience of the numbness by saying what they see and notice, with the use of a mirror, about the 'sleeping tooth' (Figure 8.4). It is also useful to tell the child's parent how long the anaesthesia may last and to indicate when the child may cautiously eat and drink again. A useful aid is a card with a clock drawn on it. On this, the clock hands are drawn so that the child knows when he/she may eat again. If a child is very hungry or thirsty and the anaesthesia has not yet worn off completely, helpful tips may be to drink through a straw and to 'eat on the other side'.

8.3   Techniques

Dentists almost exclusively use infiltration anaesthesia in children, occasionally preceded by topical anaesthesia. It seems that most dentists are reluctant to use mandibular block anaesthesia or consider this unnecessary for children. The use of intraligamentary anaesthesia is effective in children. A microprocessor-controlled form of local anaesthesia is also now available, which enables child-friendly local anaesthesia through the periodontal ligament.

8.3.1   Topical anaesthesia

The use of topical anaesthesia can offer the dentist and child more security and so contribute to a comfortable injection of anaesthetic fluid. A choice can be made between spray and ointment. Usually, the spray has a higher concentration of anaesthetic than the ointment.

If one prefers the spray, it is best to soak a cotton bud with the anaesthetic and to touch the insertion site of the needle with this. Beforehand, the mucosa must be made as dry as possible. If the cotton bud is kept in place for 2–3 minutes, the anaesthesia is usually sufficient to make the insertion of the needle unnoticeable.

Anaesthetic ointment can be applied in the same way. Again the mucosa must be made dry prior to application of the ointment. Only a small amount of ointment is required to achieve the desired result (Figure 8.5 and Box 8.4).

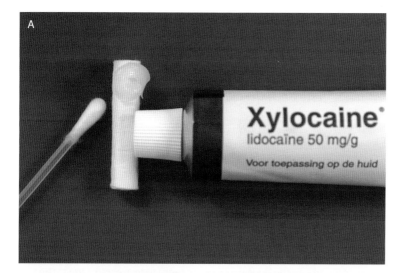

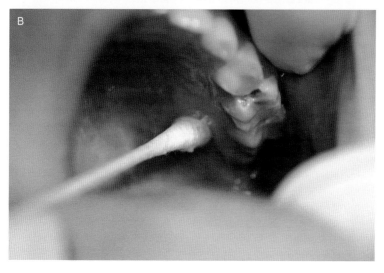

Figure 8.5 A and B
Topical anaesthesia.

Box 8.4 Colour, taste and acceptance

By mixing the ointment with cooking essences, fun colours can be made
and children will accept the taste more readily. If a child chooses out of
various colours, this implicitly means that he or she has accepted the
anaesthesia.

8.3.2   Infiltration anaesthesia

For restorations in the upper jaw in children, infiltration anaesthesia
vestibular to the respective tooth is sufficient. When two cavities in
adjacent teeth have to be treated, a single injection between both teeth
will suffice. The layer of cortical bone that covers the outside of the upper
jaw is relatively thin and porous and the anaesthetic fluid easily diffuses
to the nerve endings.

The needle is placed in the deepest point of the buccal fold with the bevel
pointed towards the bone. Because of the reabsorption of the roots of the
deciduous teeth in older children, it is sufficient to insert the needle in the
free gingiva just past the transition from the attached to the free gingiva
(Figure 8.6).

If topical anaesthesia is not being used, it is important to insert the
needle cautiously and yet determinedly, so that the pain of the insertion
is as short as possible. A certain resistance must be broken with particular
speed. The needle then sinks, as it were, through the barrier of the mucosa.

If topical anaesthesia is not being used, the needle prick can be made less
noticeable by slightly pinching the cheek, corner of the mouth or the lip
just before the moment of penetration. The child must be informed
beforehand of the slight pinch. The child is then distracted and will not or
hardly feel the needle being inserted. Perhaps even more effective is using
the suction tube in the buccal fold of the tooth to be treated. Due to the
pressure of the suction tube, the needle can be imperceptibly inserted
next to the suction tip and any spilled anaesthetic fluid will be removed
immediately.

In cases of extraction in the upper jaw, it is preferable to anaesthetise the
greater palatine nerve or the nasopalatine nerve (Figure 8.7). The palatal
anaesthesia can be given painlessly with care, especially if topical anaesthesia
is being employed. Anaesthesia of the palatine nerve can be regarded as
block anaesthesia since an anaesthetic fluid depot is created posteriorly in
the palate. This method of administration has two advantages: more teeth
on the palatal side are anaesthetised simultaneously and there is more
space under the mucosa in the transition of the vertical to the horizontal
part in the distal section of the palate. This means that less pressure is
required for the administration and the anaesthesia will be less painful.
Here it is also advantageous to place the suction tip palatinally. If the child
has been informed of the purpose of the suction tube, he/she will find the
pressure less threatening.

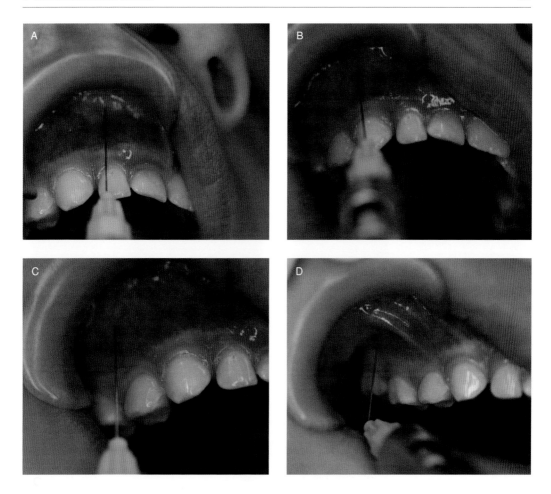

A disadvantage of block anaesthesia of the palatine nerve is that part of the soft palate is also anaesthetised, so swallowing feels strange and sometimes feelings of anxiety arise. More pressure is needed during an injection in the anterior part of the palate. This may be accompanied by pain and unexpected reactions from the child.

If deciduous teeth are being extracted, it is also possible to anaesthetise the palatal mucosa with interpapillary anaesthesia. The needle is then inserted into the papilla and 0.2 ml is slowly injected. This adequately anaesthetises the attached gingiva on the palatal side. Of course, local anaesthesia must also be applied in the mesial and distal papilla of the tooth to be extracted.

Infiltration anaesthesia in the lower jaw can only be used in young children because the structure of the cortical bone plate is not as dense. As a consequence, penetration of anaesthetic fluid after infiltration anaesthesia is relatively effective for restorative treatment of the lower incisors, deciduous canine and the first deciduous molar. The advantage of infiltration anaesthesia in the lower jaw is that a stiff lip (partially) and tongue (entirely) are avoided. However, the dentist does not know for sure

Figure 8.6 A, B, C and D
Infiltration anaesthesia.

Figure 8.7 A and B
Interpapillary and palatal
anaesthesia.

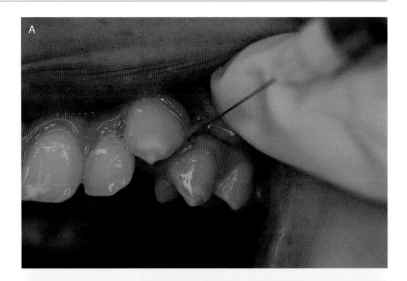

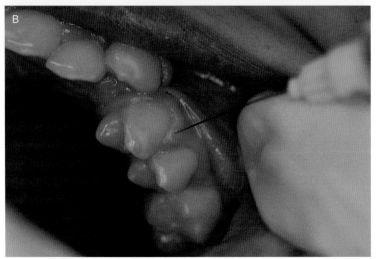

whether the anaesthesia is really effective. In strongly protesting children,
the dentist can grip a stiff lip more firmly, without the problem that pain is
the cause of the child's protest.

8.3.3 Mandibular block anaesthesia

All dental procedures in children can be carried out painlessly with
mandibular block anaesthesia. Supplementary anaesthesia of the buccal
nerve is needed for extractions, whilst the lingual nerve is automatically
anaesthetised with the mandibular injection.

There are significant differences in the size of the jaw in adults and
children. This means that for mandibular anaesthesia in children up to
12 years old, the injection must be given at the level of the occlusal plane.
The injection should be given less deeply for children, because the

foramen, seen from the front, is located at one-third of the mandibular ramus width.

Children generally find mandibular anaesthesia a far-reaching experience due to the numb cheek, lip and tingling tongue. If the dental treatment plan allows it, it is therefore sensible to start with those treatments for which infiltration anaesthesia is sufficient.

The technique of mandibular block anaesthesia hardly differs for children and adults. The child is asked to open the mouth wide. With thumb and index finger, the dentist seeks respectively the anterior and posterior sides of the mandibular ascending branch (Figure 8.8). Measured from the front, the mandibular foramen lies at one-third of the imaginary line between the index finger and thumb.

A slightly better grip on the lower jaw and a better fixation of the head are possible by a little modification of this method. The position of the

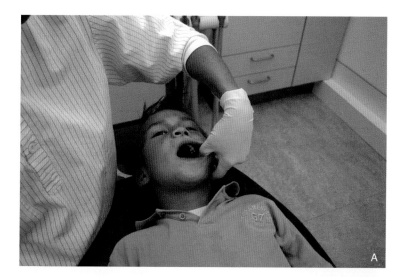

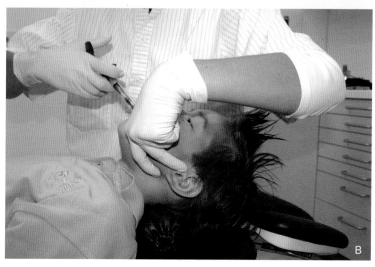

Figure 8.8 A and B
Mandibular block anaesthesia.

thumb remains the same, but the index finger is placed on the head of the mandible and the ring finger is placed in the corner of the jaw, while the middle finger is placed in the middle of the back side of the mandibular ascending branch. Working in the left mandibula, the ring finger is placed on the head of the mandibula and the index finger in the corner.

8.3.4   Intraligamental anaesthesia

For intraligamental anaesthesia along the periodontal ligament the anaesthetic fluid diffuses through small openings in the alveolar wall to the intraossal space and from there the nerve is blocked. The adjacent mucosa will also be numbed.

The intraligamental technique is an effective method for achieving analgesia for teeth and molars of the deciduous dentition as well as for permanent teeth (Figure 8.9). With the use of intraligamental

Figure 8.9 A, B and C

Intraligamentary anaesthesia.

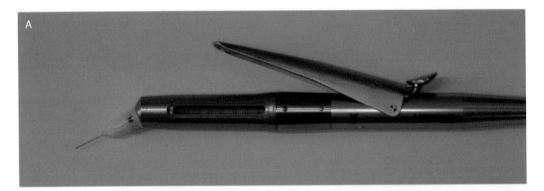

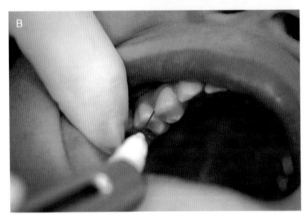

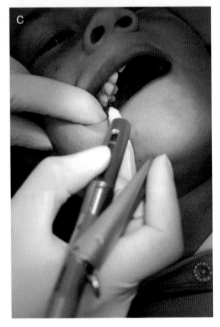

anaesthesia, for example Citoject® or Paroject®, a high pressure develops in the periodontal ligament. When this technique is used in the deciduous dentition, in theory this could cause developmental problems in tooth buds of the permanent teeth. If some time is taken between each 'click' of the intraligamental syringe, the build-up of pressure in the periodontal ligament will be limited.

8.3.5   Microprocessor-controlled anaesthesia

Besides manual cartridge syringes, nowadays microprocessor-controlled local anaesthesia can also be used. An example is The Wand® (Milestone) which was introduced in 1997 (Figure 8.10). Because of its design, which bears no resemblance to the classical cartridge syringe, this apparatus is especially suited to those children and adults who have a fear of dentists.

A sterile and disposable hand piece, in which standard anaesthetic cartridges can be inserted, is supplied for the application of anaesthetic fluid. The Wand® is activated by the foot. The step motor of the pump unit ensures that the pressure and the flow rate of the injection fluid remain low. After the injection, the step motor backs up so that there is no leakage of anaesthetic fluid.

Figure 8.10 A, B and C
Microprocessor-controlled anaesthesia.

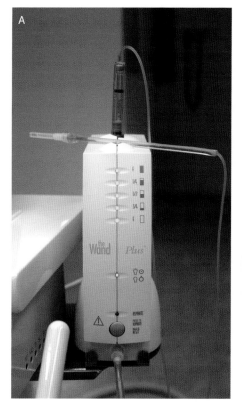
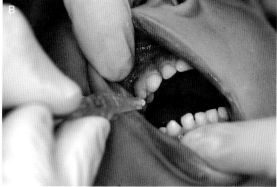
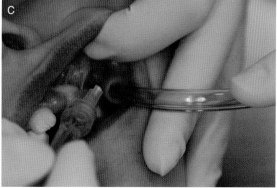

In addition to the use of infiltration and block anaesthesia, intraossal anaesthesia can be given along the periodontal ligament, the incisive foramen and the foramina at the level of the maxillary premolar roots. The hand piece is held in a pen grip, so that it is possible to lean on and allow a steady and precise insertion of the needle.

The injection is given on the mesiobuccal and distobuccal line angle of the tooth. With the use of anaesthesia along the periodontal ligament, dental treatments on both sides of the mandibula can be performed in a single session, without the lip and tongue being anaesthetised bilaterally.

8.3.6 Amount of anaesthetic fluid for children

No absolute numbers can be given for the required amount of anaesthetic fluid. Table 8.1 provides the maximum dosage for children. The amount of anaesthetic fluid required for a painless preparation or extraction within a quadrant rarely exceeds the volume of two cartridges. Therefore the maximum dose for children is not easily exceeded.

Table 8.1	Maximum dosage of some frequently used local anaesthetics for healthy children.					
Weight of child	Articaine 4%		Lidocaine 2%		Prilocaine 3%	
kg	mg[1]	cartridges[2]	mg[1]	cartridges[2]	mg[1]	cartridges[2]
5–10	25	0.3	22	0.6	30	0.5
10–15	50	0.7	44	1.2	60	1.1
15–20	75	1.0	66	1.8	90	1.6
20–25	100	1.3	88	2.4	120	2.2
25–30	125	1.7	110	3.0	150	2.7
30–35	150	2.0	132	3.6	180	3.3
35–40	175	2.4	154	4.2	210	3.8
40–45	200	2.7	176	4.8	240	4.4

[1]The maximum dosage indicated is for healthy children. This maximum also depends on individual differences, the way the anaesthetic is administered and the extent of vascularisation of the tissue.

[2]The number of cartridges is based on cartridges with a volume of 1.8 ml.

This table is based on Malamed, S.F. (2004) *Handbook of Local Anesthesia*, Mosby, St. Louis.

8.4　Observation of the child

It is important to keep an eye on the child continuously during and after giving local anaesthesia. Verification that the anaesthetic 'works' increases the confidence of the child. Explanation of the procedure is essential and must be adapted to the child's age. The child may, for example, notice the sharp point of the dental probe on a finger, while in the anaesthetised mouth the child just notices pressure of the same probe or even nothing at all. It is important that the child can watch the procedure in a mirror.

8.5　Complications of mandibular block anaesthesia

Despite the extensive information given to young patients and their parents, there is a chance that children may bite their numb and later tingling lip. This may cause a traumatic ulcer to occur (Figure 8.11). The danger of a bite wound is greatest if the treatment has taken place around noon. Children are then usually hungry and will start to eat before the anaesthesia has completely subsided. In such situations it is better for the dentist to advise the child to eat before the dental treatment. Another cause of bite wounds is that children wish to test if the anaesthesia is still working or whether it has worn off completely.

Figure 8.11 A, B and C
Complications of mandibular
block anaesthesia in children.

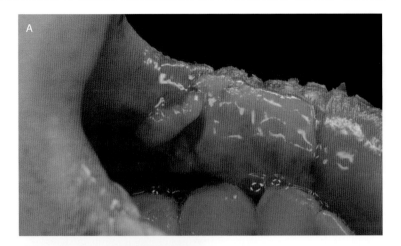

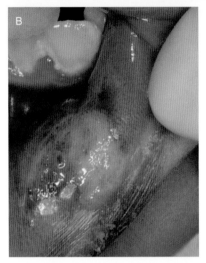

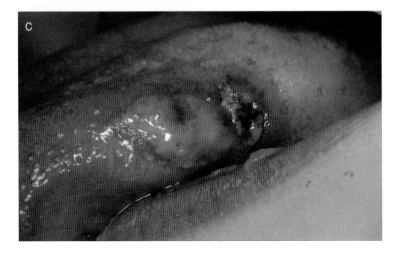

9 Local complications

H.P. van den Akker

Local anaesthesia is frequently used in dentistry and seldom leads to serious local complications. Nevertheless, it is of great importance to be aware of the causes of each local complication and – if necessary – to implement correct treatment. The patient must be informed extensively and, if necessary, be reassured. The incident must also be recorded in detail in the patient's file. This is especially important if there is a chance of prolonged or even permanent symptoms.

9.1 Needle breakage

Since the introduction of modern disposable needles, needle breakage is a rare complication. Nevertheless, even these needles have a small chance of breaking, especially with mandibular block anaesthesia and tuberosity anaesthesia. This risk increases if the needle is repeatedly bent to facilitate the entrance into the area to be injected. The unexpected movements of a scared patient, such as a sudden jerk of the head, grabbing or moving away the dentist's hand or suddenly closing the mouth, can also lead to this serious complication. Changing the direction of an incorrectly inserted needle also increases the risk of needle breakage. In such a situation, it is sensible to pull back the needle almost completely and then insert it again in the correct direction.

If the needle does break and the proximal part of the needle is still sticking out of the mucosa, the end may be taken with tweezers or mosquito artery forceps and cautiously removed. However, if the broken part of the needle is no longer visible the patient must be referred quickly to an oral and maxillofacial surgeon in a well-equipped hospital (Box 9.1). In the meantime, the patient must be instructed not to talk and to swallow as little as possible, since such movements may allow the needle to move deeper into the tissues.

Box 9.1

Prevention of needle breakage:
1 Use a 27-gauge 35 mm needle for mandibular block.
2 Do not bend the needle repeatedly and not immediately next to the mandrel.
3 Avoid inserting up to the hilt of the needle.
4 Do not change direction of the needle while injecting.

What the dentist should do if the broken needle is visible:
• Try to remove the needle with a fine haemostat.

What the dentist should do if the broken needle is not visible:
• Mark the place of insertion of the needle with a waterproof marker.
• Inform the patient and advise to avoid jaw movements.
• Contact the oral and maxillofacial surgeon immediately.
• Contact your defence union and discuss the case with colleagues.

What the oral and maxillofacial surgeon should do:
• Arrange immediate assessment of the patient.
• Arrange immediate radiographic examination (OPG and CT-scan).
• Discuss treatment modalities with the patient, parent or carer.
• Arrange surgical exploration.

9.2   Pain during administration

Even during a calm and slow injection, the patient sometimes feels some discomfort or a burning sensation when the needle is introduced through the soft tissues. An increase in tissue pressure from injecting too quickly or injecting a too-large volume is unpleasant for the patient and must of course be avoided. A pronounced pain sensation is, however, usually the result of unintentionally pricking an anatomical structure, e.g. a tendon or muscle, the periosteum, a nerve or blood vessel.

Pricking the periosteum is usually the result of an incorrect position of the bevel of the needle. The bevel should be placed parallel to the bone surface, to avoid the sharp point of the needle pricking the tight and highly innervated periosteum and tearing it away from the underlying bone. During the administration of mandibular block anaesthesia the inferior alveolar nerve or the lingual nerve can be inadvertently touched. The patient will experience this as a shot of pain or a sensation like an 'electric' shock in the lower jaw or the tongue and will react by suddenly pulling away the head. If this occurs, the needle must be pulled back slightly and, if necessary, the direction of insertion must be altered before injecting the anaesthetic fluid. Such contact of the needle with a nerve does not automatically mean that sensation disorders will occur, but the patient must be informed of the possibility and, if necessary, should be regularly checked. It is good to realise that the occurrence is not an indication of a poor injection technique, but simply a risk that is inevitably related to the administration of block anaesthesia.

A shot of pain may also occur if the artery wall is touched, resulting in the phenomenon of 'blanching' (see Section 9.7).

9.3   Insufficient anaesthesia

The most prevalent causes of failure of local anaesthesia are an incorrect injection technique and an injection into inflamed tissue or a blood vessel. For maximal anaesthesia, the anaesthetic fluid must be deposited near the nerve or, in infiltration anaesthesia, as close as possible to the bone surface in the apex region of the element that is to be anaesthetised. In the case of block anaesthesia in the lower jaw, the vertical aspect of the position of the mandibular foramen must be taken into account. If the direction of the needle is too low and the anaesthetic fluid is injected below the level of the foramen, there will be no anaesthetic effect, partly due to the effect of gravity. If infiltration anaesthesia is given in an inflamed area, the local anaesthetic will be less effective due to the lower pH of the tissue. In that case, adequate anaesthesia can be achieved by infiltration at a distance or by block anaesthesia.

During the insertion of the needle it is important to take care that the slanted part of the needle (the 'bevel') points to the tooth that is to be anaesthetised. Otherwise the fluid will move in the wrong direction, to a place far from its goal. Since diffusion must occur over a larger distance, this could lead to insufficient or even lack of anaesthesia. The same applies if the anaesthetic fluid is deposited in a muscle due to incorrect position of the needle. In that case, diffusion of the fluid is also hindered by the barrier of muscle tissue. An intravascular injection, resulting in injection of local anaesthetic into the bloodstream, is another cause of insufficient anaesthesia. A diffusion problem caused by a local haematoma can also play a role here. Less frequent causes are individual anatomical variations, for example, in the density of the cortical bone or divergent nerve pathways. A good example of the latter is an occasional accessory branch of the inferior alveolar nerve that first runs ventrally and then only disappears into the bone at the front of the ascending branch. This can explain pain experienced in the lower jaw despite apparently well-placed mandibular block anaesthesia.

9.4   Excessive spread of anaesthesia

Injecting a local anaesthetic into the mouth can sometimes have an unintentional effect on neighbouring nerves. The most obvious example is paresis or paralysis of the motor facial nerve after mandibular block anaesthesia. If this occurs, the patient is unable to close the eye at will, the movement of the lower half of the face is distorted, the nasolabial fold is absent and the corner of the mouth droops.

This complication is caused by an incorrect path of the needle, which is inserted too deep and too far dorsally, and the local anaesthetic is deposited retromandibular in the deep lobe of the parotid gland. This can be avoided in mandibular anaesthesia by injecting the fluid only after contact has been made with the bone on the medial side of the ascending part of the mandibula.

Though the occurrence of facial paralysis is disconcerting for both patient and dentist, it is necessary to realise that the phenomenon is temporary. The function of the nerve will return as soon as the effect of the local anaesthetic has worn off. Because the patient is not able to blink during the paralysis, there is a risk of the eye drying out and being damaged. Damage can be avoided by placing tape over the closed eyelid or wearing an eye patch.

Dental local anaesthesia can sometimes also have undesirable effects on the eyeball, the eye muscles and surrounding soft tissues. Such complications have been described both following an injection in the maxillary tuberosity region and after mandibular block anaesthesia. Intra-arterial injections of a local anaesthetic into the inferior or superior alveolar artery or pricking an artery vessel wall, causing a traumatic stimulation of the sympathetic fibres that run through it, may cause a spasm of the vessels that supply blood to the orbital tissues. If the injection pressure during intra-arterial injection exceeds the arterial blood pressure, the normal centripetal blood flow may reverse (retrograde flow) and the local anaesthetic may reach the orbit via the maxillary artery and an anastomosis between the middle meningeal artery and the ophthalmic artery. A vasospasm of the ophthalmic artery or its branch to the retina (central retinal artery) can lead to ipsilateral reduction in vision or even blindness. However, with the use of modern local anaesthetics these vision distortions are almost always reversible.

Paralysis of the cranial nerves that innervate the external eye muscles may also occur. This (rare) complication usually occurs after an injection in the maxillary tuberosity region. Because there is no complete separation of the retromaxillary area and the orbit, the anaesthetic fluid may diffuse from the site of injection into the orbit. In the orbit the effect of the local anaesthetic may cause double vision (diplopia) or the drooping of the upper eyelid (ptosis), through vasoconstriction or interference with the nerve conduction.

The Horner syndrome is a special complication, whereby pupil dilation, ptosis and absence of lacrimal secretion are observed as a result of a unilateral block of the cervical sympathetic fibres. This is probably caused by bleeding due to perforation of an external carotid artery branch, so that the local anaesthetic has reached the sympathetic ganglion stellatum.

All the above-mentioned symptoms disappear within a few hours, as soon as the effect of the local anaesthetic has worn off. During this period, the patient must be discouraged explicitly from driving or otherwise using the roads, considering the increased risk of an accident.

9.5   Iatrogenic damage and self-inflicted damage of anaesthetised tissues

The local anaesthetics used in dentistry often anaesthetise not only the teeth, but also the soft tissues that are innervated by the respective nerve. An example of this is the numb lip after mandibular block anaesthesia or following infiltration anaesthesia near the upper front teeth. Anaesthetised soft tissues may be damaged accidentally without the patient noticing, either by the dentist performing the treatment or the patient him/herself. Examples of iatrogenic damage by the dentist are a drill that shoots out, or tissue caught by the incorrect placing of a hook or extraction forceps. Burn wounds may also occur, caused by an overheated dental hand piece. Because the effect of the local anaesthetic has not yet worn off after the dental treatment, there is a chance that the patient will bite the numb lip, cheek or tongue. Other possible causes of self-inflicted damage are burn wounds caused by smoking or consumption of hot drinks or food. This may result in an ulcer or even disfiguring tissue damage. This risk is greater with children, people with learning difficulties and patients suffering from dementia. The companions of these patients must be warned of the possibilities of such injuries and must be advised to keep a careful eye on them during the remaining anaesthetic period, and not to allow them to smoke, eat or drink.

9.6   Persistent sensitivity disorders

The occurrence of a persistent sensitivity disorder in the innervation area of a nerve is usually the result of surgical treatment, such as a wisdom tooth extraction. Only very rarely is it a complication of the administration of local anaesthesia. In that case, it is almost always the inferior alveolar nerve or the lingual nerve that is affected, owing to damage during mandibular block anaesthesia. The symptoms vary from a reduced or complete loss of feeling (hypaesthesia or anaesthesia) to abnormal sensations, such as itching or tingling (paraesthesia) in the respective area. Only very occasionally it may lead to a chronic pain syndrome.

The occurrence of sensitivity disorders and their duration are determined by the extent of the damage to the nerve. If the needle is immediately removed after direct contact with a nerve, there will be no symptoms once the anaesthesia has worn off. The case is different if nerve fibres are directly damaged by deep penetration of the needle or if the nerve is, as it were, blown up by an intraneural injection under high pressure. A haemorrhage within the nerve sheath, resulting in compression of the fibres, may also cause a prolonged conduction disorder. A change of symptoms within a few weeks to months, for example a transition from anaesthesia to paraesthesia, is a good sign and indicates recovery of the nerve function. If, however, the sensibility disorder persists unaltered for more than 3–6 months, the chance of recovery decreases and the final prognosis is negative. Then it is sensible to refer the patient to an oral and maxillofacial surgeon to evaluate the situation and to discuss possible treatment.

9.7   Skin paleness ('blanching')

Directly following – and even during – an injection in the buccal fold of the upper jaw near the premolars and molars, it is possible that a sudden blanching of the skin may occur in the respective half of the face, especially in the cheek and the area around the eye (see Figure 9.1). Occasionally ischaemic areas may also occur in the oral mucosa at some distance from the injection point. The phenomenon may also occur during the administration of mandibular block anaesthesia. Often this is accompanied by shooting pain in the affected area and by reduced vision. The symptoms generally disappear quickly over the next few minutes to half an hour.

The cause is probably a prick to the artery wall, resulting in traumatic stimulation of the orthosympathetic nerve fibres in the artery wall, causing a vessel spasm. The impulse is then carried along the blood vessel, leading to vasoconstriction in the peripheral supply area of the artery. A direct effect on the vessel wall of the vasoconstrictor during local anaesthesia may also play a role in this.

Figure 9.1
'Blanching'.

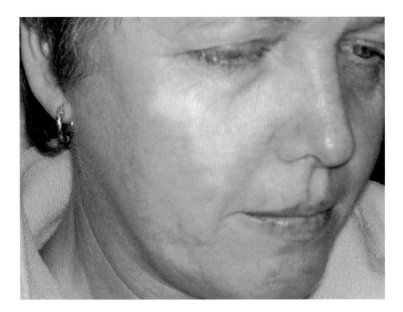

9.8   Tissue necrosis

The occurrence of tissue necrosis in the injection area is a well known – but thankfully rare – complication of local anaesthesia administration. This undesirable effect is mainly observed on the hard palate (Figure 9.2), partly

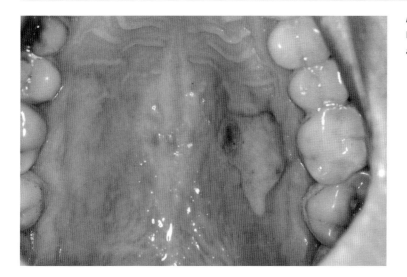

Figure 9.2
Palatal mucosa necrosis after administration of anaesthesia.

caused by the toughness of the palatal mucosa and its sturdy attachment to the underlying bone. The most probable explanation for this complication is local ischaemia, caused by one or more factors. These include an excessively high injection pressure, the injection of too much anaesthetic fluid into the tight tissue or a vasoconstrictor-induced narrowing of the small palatine end arteries. Usually this results in a superficial necrotic ulcer of the mucosa, which heals spontaneously within a few weeks. Good oral hygiene and rinsing with a chlorhexidine solution several times a day will boost the healing process. In exceptional cases, such as when the periosteum is raised by a subperiosteal injection, the underlying bone may be exposed and a painful bone infection may develop. Necrosis of the palate can usually be avoided by injecting a maximum of 0.25 ml of anaesthetic fluid at very low pressure in the transition area from the horizontal hard palate to the alveolar process.

9.9   Haematoma formation and trismus

A haematoma develops if, during insertion of the needle, a blood vessel is penetrated and blood leaks into the surrounding tissues. If the perforated vessel is large and the surrounding soft tissues are loose, a relatively large swelling may occur. At the usual injection sites, dental local anaesthesia has a low risk of a clinically relevant haematoma. However, complications of this kind are possible, particularly with mandibular block anaesthesia and injections into the area of the maxillary tuberosity and the floor of the mouth.

A haematoma resulting from block anaesthesia at the point of the mandibular foramen may develop between the medial side of the mandibular ascending branch and the medial pterygoid muscle. This can lead to swelling in the pharyngeal arch area and the occurrence of slight trismus. The trismus is usually noticed only a few hours after the injection and will usually disappear within 1–2 weeks if the patient performs daily mouth exercises. An increase of the trismus indicates secondary infection of the haematoma and requires immediate antibiotic treatment. Trismus can also occur if a haematoma develops in the medial pterygoid muscle due to incorrect needle direction in mandibular block anaesthesia. As a result of scarring, this can lead to long-term difficulty in opening the mouth, which usually requires intensive physiotherapy.

In tuberosity anaesthesia a haematoma may develop in the retromaxillary area due to a perforation of the pterygoid venous plexus. Externally, this becomes visible as a rapidly increasing swelling of the cheek around the zygoma. Subsequently, a slight form of trismus may also occur.

Haematomas may cause the patient a lot of discomfort and may cause embarrassment to the dentist, but the swelling restricts itself and usually does not require extensive treatment. Applying immediate pressure, possibly with an elasticated bandage, and applying ice intermittently during the first 4–6 hours may help to restrict the extent of the swelling. The swelling and subsequent blue–yellow discolouration of the skin diminish slowly. Of course, it is important to correctly inform the patient about the incident and the expected course. The patient must be advised to contact the dentist if symptoms arise that may indicate a secondary infection. Examples of this are increasing swelling or trismus and/or fever or general malaise.

9.10   Infection

Although every intra-oral injection with a sterile disposable needle will introduce micro-organisms of the normal oral flora into the tissue, this rarely leads to clinical infection in healthy people. However, in immunocompromised patients the dentist must consider disinfecting the injection area prior to injecting by locally applying an antiseptic or with a chlorhexidine mouthwash. Of course, the needle must never be inserted through an infection infiltrate or an abscess, since this considerably increases the risk of dislodging micro-organisms and aggravation of the infection. In such cases, anaesthesia must be given at a distance (block anaesthesia).

If a secondary infection arises in a haematoma that has emerged during the administration of a local anaesthetic, there is a chance that an abscess will develop. This mainly applies to haematomas in the pterygomandibular space, in the retromaxillary area and in the floor of the mouth. If the haematoma is infected the slight trismus already present will increase in severity rapidly, and occasionally this happens in such a way that after a few days the mouth can no longer be opened at all. In the case of an abscess in the pterygomandibular space there is hardly any external swelling present, at most a slight swelling around the mandibular angle.

There may, however, be serious pain during palpation just inside the jaw corner. If the trismus allows, an intra-oral investigation may establish in the pharyngeal arch area the presence of a swelling that is painful during palpation. Besides fever and general malaise, a further spreading of the infection may result in increasing pain and problems with swallowing.

An abscess from a haematoma in the retromaxillary space can spread to adjacent spaces, increasing the risk of venous thrombophlebitis with intracranial complications. If medical symptoms indicate the development of an infection infiltrate or an abscess, the patient must be treated with antibiotics, possibly in combination with incision and drainage of the relevant area.

10 Systemic complications

H.S. Brand, A.L. Frankhuijzen and J.F.M. Fennis

When employed correctly, local anaesthetics are remarkably safe agents, though unwanted systemic reactions may still occur after administration of a local anaesthetic. Dentists should prevent these side effects as much as possible, recognise them at an early stage and treat them adequately.

10.1 Introduction

Few data are available about the frequency of side effects of local anaesthetics. Since hundreds of thousands of cartridges are used worldwide every day and complications are hardly reported, it seems evident that local anaesthetics – in low doses and administered with a (self-) aspirating syringe – are remarkably safe. Psychogenic reactions such as vasovagal collapse and hyperventilation are the most frequently occurring side effects.

10.2 Vasovagal collapse

The most common systemic complications following local anaesthesia occur due to emotional reactions to the way the anaesthesia is administered. Psychogenic anticipation of the possible pain of the injection can activate the parasympathetic nervous system as well as inhibit the orthosympathetic nervous system. This causes a reduction in heart rate and dilatation of the arterioles in muscles, inducing a temporary shortness of blood flow to the brain.

The patient suffering from vasovagal collapse looks pale, perspires and may lose consciousness. In addition to the loss of consciousness, sometimes clonic cramps occur which resemble an epileptic convulsion. The duration of the collapse is usually short lived. With an (imminent) vasovagal collapse, the dental chair should be placed in the Trendelenburg position, with the body flat on the back and the feet higher than the head, whereupon consciousness will return in a short time.

10.3   Hyperventilation syndrome

Fear of injection of a local anaesthetic can also serve as a trigger for abnormally fast and deep breathing, reducing the level of carbon dioxide in the blood (pCO_2). The pH of the blood increases and the concentration of ionised calcium decreases. Muscle contractions develop, which can present periorally. Additionally, the patient perceives a tingling sensation in the hands and feet. Sometimes the patient feels light-headed and can experience chest pressure.

Treatment consists of reassurance, and asking the patient to breathe into a paper bag. Rebreathing expired air will increase the pCO_2 and usually resolves the condition rapidly. If possible, the dentist should 'dictate' the correct breathing frequency to the patient.

Supplying accurate information to the patient about the administration of local anaesthesia, combined with fear-reducing treatment, reduces the risk of hyperventilation and vasovagal collapse.

10.4   Toxicity

It is conceivable that, as a result of the oral administration of a local anaesthetic, toxic concentrations may develop elsewhere in the body. An accidental intravascular injection can cause a short-lived toxic concentration of the anaesthetic in the blood. An increased resorption rate – which may exist in inflamed tissue with increased blood flow – could also result in unexpectedly high levels of anaesthetic in the blood. Comparable toxic effects may be observed if topical anaesthetics are sprayed directly onto (inflamed) mucosa. An overdose is usually the result of using a higher dose than the maximum allowed, generally caused by repeat injections. Most cases of overdose occur in children.

The toxicity of amide anaesthetics is reciprocally related to their degradation rate in the liver. Prilocaine is metabolised most rapidly and is therefore the least toxic amide anaesthetic. In addition, prilocaine has a high degree of binding to tissue proteins (a large distribution volume), so potentially a toxic concentration is reached less rapidly.

Table 10.1 presents the maximum dosages for adults of some regularly used local anaesthetics. Of course, these values must be individualised based on the patient's body weight and medical history (Box 10.1). Patients with reduced detoxification and elimination, such as individuals with severe liver insufficiency or kidney failure, are at increased risk of overdose. Possible interaction with other medications should also be considered, as some pharmaceuticals lower the threshold for side effects of local anaesthetics (see Chapter 11).

10.4.1   Effects on the central nervous system

The local anaesthetics used in dentistry can cross the blood–brain barrier easily because of their lipophilic nature. Under physiological conditions,

Table 10.1	Maximum dosages of frequently used local anaesthetics (in milligrams for healthy individuals of 70 kg).	
	Without adrenaline	*With adrenaline*
Articaine	400	500
Bupivacaine	75	150
Lidocaine	300	500
Mepivacaine	375	400
Prilocaine	400	600

Box 10.1 A sensible dentist calculates in milligrams

The concentration of a local anaesthetic in the cartridge is expressed as a percentage, while the added vasoconstrictor is expressed as a ratio. Since the concentrations of local anaesthetic and/or vasoconstrictor may differ per cartridge, it is necessary to be able to convert these into milligrams.

1. Dose of local anaesthetic (articaine with adrenaline)
    Maximum dose of articaine in milligrams:
        7 mg/kg × 70 kg = 490 mg
    Concentration in cartridge: 4% = 40 mg/ml
        490 mg/(40 mg/ml) = 12.25 ml
        1 cartridge = 1.7 ml
    Maximum dose of articaine in cartridges:
        12.25 ml/1.7 ml = 7 cartridges
2. Dose of vasoconstrictor (articaine with adrenaline)
    Maximum dose of adrenaline in micrograms:
        3 µg/kg × 70 kg = 210 µg
    Concentration in cartridge: 1:200,000 g/ml
        $= 5 \times 10^{-6}$ g/ml
        = 5 µg/ml
    1 cartridge = 1.7 ml = 1.7 × 5 = 8.5 µg adrenaline
    Maximum dose of articaine = 7 cartridges = 7 × 8.5 µg = 59.5 µg adrenaline.

This is more than a factor of three less than the maximum dose of adrenaline. Therefore with regard to toxicity, the maximum dose is seven cartridges of anaesthetic. This also applies to articaine with the same concentration of local anaesthetic, but a dose of adrenaline that is twice as high (1:100,000).

the central nervous system receives both inhibitory and stimulatory impulses. Since the inhibitory tonus prevails under normal conditions, an inhibition of the central nervous system by a toxic concentration of anaesthetic will manifest as an excitation. The patient will feel dizzy and complain of tinnitus (ringing in the ears). With increased excitation, the patient becomes afraid and trembling. Breathing quickens, blood pressure rises and heartbeat frequency increases. The patient develops facial twitches and seizures may arise. The severity of the symptoms correlates with the level of anaesthetic in the blood. After a further increase in the level of anaesthetic in the blood, a depression of the central nervous system develops which reduces consciousness. Breathing frequency decreases and may even progress to respiratory arrest. The circulation becomes insufficient and ultimately the patient may go into a coma (Box 10.2).

After intravascular injection, the toxic effects on the central nervous system will manifest very rapidly (within 1 minute). Distribution of the anaesthetic within the body decreases the concentration rapidly, and the toxic effects disappear soon too. With an overdose, the effects on the central nervous system develop more gradually, usually after 5–15 minutes, and the symptoms will persist much longer.

Box 10.2

A feeling of light-headedness is an obvious initial symptom of central toxicity. It is assumed that to a great extent this is caused by central cholinergic stimulation. These initial clinical signs are hard to distinguish from vasovagal stimulation.

The excitation phase may partially be the result of an apparent inhibition of inhibitory neurons in the central nervous system or a non-selective inhibition during a predominant inhibition of the central nervous system. Whereas almost all local anaesthetics have inherent vasodilatory activity, an initial vasoconstriction may occur by displacing Ca^{2+} from the cell membrane. This has been reported frequently with prilocaine and mepivacaine. At higher concentrations of anaesthetic, a more generalised inhibition of neurons will occur. This general depression of the central nervous system may ultimately result in loss of consciousness, reduced breathing frequency, a certain inhibition of the autonomic ganglia and finally cardiovascular collapse.

10.4.2   Cardiovascular effects

Since the heart is much less sensitive to overdoses of anaesthetic than the brain, cardiotoxic effects usually manifest much later than the effects on the central nervous system. Cardiologists even use lidocaine in plasma concentrations of 1–3 µg/ml for the acute treatment of heart rhythm disturbances. Higher concentrations of the anaesthetic (5–10 µg/ml) lead to an inhibition of the action potential conduction in the heart. This results in decreased frequency of the heartbeat and reduced contraction strength of the myocardium. At concentrations over 10 µg/ml the severity of these effects increases, as a result of which ultimately even loss of circulation may occur.

The cardiotoxicity of local anaesthetics is not only concentration dependent, but also related to the strength of the anaesthetic effect. Lidocaine has the smallest negative effect on the contraction strength of the heart muscle. With more potent local anaesthetics, such as bupivacaine, there is less difference between the dose that has toxic effects on the central nervous system and the dose resulting in cardiovascular toxicity.

10.4.3   Treatment of toxic reactions

The treatment of an overdose of local anaesthetic depends on the severity of the reaction. In most cases, the clinical signs are mild and transient, and do not require specific treatment since the concentration of the anaesthetic in the brain and heart will drop rapidly due to degradation and blood redistribution in the body. The patient should be reassured, and breathing and circulation monitored continuously. If convulsions occur, arms and legs should be protected against injuries.

In the very rare situation that the heart contraction reducing effect of local anaesthetic induces an insufficient circulation, the patient should be transferred to the emergency department of a hospital under administration of oxygen and, if necessary, resuscitation.

10.5   Systemic effects of vasoconstrictors

Signs of intoxication caused by added vasoconstrictors are rare, and will only cause complications after intravascular injection. An increase in the concentration of adrenaline in the blood can cause a considerable increase in blood pressure and heart rate (Box 10.3). At higher levels of adrenaline in the blood, feelings of fear and restlessness develop. The patient feels tremulous, looks pale and begins to perspire heavily. Heart rhythm disorders are also among the possible side effects.

Toxic effects, such as an increase in blood pressure, have also been attributed to felypressin. However, these effects usually only occur with doses that are five- to ten-fold the maximum recommended amount. For adults, the maximum dosage of felypressin is 5.4 µg and of adrenaline is 200 µg.

The risk of intravascular administration of a vasoconstrictor can be minimised by using (self-) aspirating syringes. In addition, one should realise that pain due to insufficient anaesthesia may result in a high endogenous release of adrenaline in the circulation. The risk of this is at least as high as the risks of a low dose of added vasoconstrictor. Besides,

---

Box 10.3

The vasoconstriction by adrenaline is the result of a stimulation of α_1-adrenergic receptors on the smooth muscles of blood vessels. In the blood vessels of skeletal tissues adrenaline also has a vasodilatory effect by binding to β_2-adrenergic receptors, which decrease the diastolic blood pressure. The strong effect of adrenaline on β_1-adrenergic receptors in the heart stimulates the heart action by increasing the contractile force (positive ionotropic effect), increasing the conduction velocity in the heart (positive dromotropic effect) and increasing the heart frequency (positive chronotropic effect), which can raise the systolic blood pressure substantially. Extrasystoles can also occur and, with high doses of adrenaline, even ventricular fibrillation or a cardiac arrest. A rapid increase in systolic blood pressure may result in a throbbing headache.

---

the addition of a vasoconstrictor is a protective measure against the toxicity of the anaesthetic: it delays the resorption of the anaesthetic and avoids the necessity of repeat injections during treatment.

10.6   Allergic reactions

In the past, ester anaesthetics frequently led to allergic reactions. The PABA analogues that arise during the degradation of ester anaesthetics are responsible for this. With the current use of amide anaesthetics, allergic reactions are extremely rare. Considering the biochemical structure of adrenaline and the presence of it in the body, an allergic reaction to this vasoconstrictor seems to be unlikely. Felypressin is a foreign peptide, which, at least theoretically, may induce an allergic reaction. Hypersensitivity reactions after the administration of local anaesthesia are usually attributed to the added preservatives and antioxidants. Since these days the preservatives methylparaben and propylparaben are hardly used anymore in cartridges of local anaesthetics, the antioxidant bisulphite is probably the most frequent cause of an allergic reaction after the administration of local anaesthesia.

Essentially, two types of allergic reactions may arise: the immediate hypersensitivity reaction (type I reaction) and the delayed hypersensitivity reaction (type IV reaction).

10.6.1   Immediate hypersensitivity reactions

IgE-antibodies on mast cells play a central role in an immediate hypersensitivity (anaphylactic) reaction. Patients may have developed IgE-antibodies against a component of the local anaesthetic. When this agent is administered again in these patients, it will bind to the IgE-molecules on the surface of the mast cells. This immediately activates the mast cells, which release histamine into the surrounding tissues, which causes vasodilatation, increased vascular permeability and smooth muscle contraction. The reactions occur within 1 hour after the injection of the local anaesthetic; extreme reactions may even develop within 1 minute.

Clinical signs may differ in severity. Locally, redness, itching and oedema may develop. Laryngeal and glottic oedemas are associated with the risk of suffocation. Severe reactions may lead to hypotension, tachycardia, loss of consciousness and – in rare cases – anaphylactic shock. In an anaphylactic shock, the patient does not look pale but pink, due to the generalised vasodilatation.

10.6.2 Delayed hypersensitivity reactions

A delayed hypersensitivity reaction is dependent on sensibilised T-lymphocytes. At renewed contact with the allergen, the T-lymphocytes will be activated and release specific proteins (cytokines). This induces a local inflammatory reaction with concomitant tissue damage that is associated with redness and swelling. A delayed hypersensitivity reaction to the anaesthetic can also manifest as a lichenoid reaction (Box 10.4). With delayed hypersensitivity to an injected local anaesthetic, the patient usually complains of painful, burning mucosa. Delayed hypersensitivity reactions develop slowly over 24–72 hours, although in cases of severe sensibilisation the first signs may present after several hours.

Box 10.4

The frequent application of a local anaesthetic on the skin may induce sensibilisation, leading to the development of contact eczema, a type IV hypersensitivity reaction. In the past, when local anaesthetics of the ester type were still used in dentistry regularly, contact eczema was frequently observed on the fingers of dentists and dental assistants due to spilling of injection fluid. The amide type anaesthetics used today are weak allergens. Nowadays, allergic contact eczema of dentists is usually caused by latex gloves or the ingredients of composites and adhesives.

10.6.3 Treatment of allergic reactions

An anaphylactic shock is a life-threatening situation. A patient who develops an extensive allergic reaction within minutes of the administration of a local anaesthetic, with hypotension, tachycardia, respiratory difficulties and/or loss of consciousness, should be treated immediately. First, the patient should be placed in the Trendelenburg position. Adrenaline must be injected intramuscularly to forestall the decrease in blood pressure. Next, both an antihistamine and a

Table 10.2	Treatment of an anaphylactic reaction.

- Terminate dental treatment

- Place the patient in the Trendelenburg position (head lower than legs)

Further treatment depends on the severity of the clinical signs

If the reaction is limited to the skin:

- Administer an oral antihistamine, e.g. one tablet of 10 mg cetirizine (Zyrtec®) or one tablet of 10 mg loratadine (Claritin®)

With severe systemic signs:

- Inject 0.5–1.0 ml adrenaline (1 ampoule containing 1 mg/ml) IM in the triceps of the upper arm, and repeat if necessary after 5 minutes

- Similarly, inject 2 ml clemastine (Tavegil®; 1 ampoule of 2 ml containing 1 mg/ml)

- Similarly, inject a corticosteroid, e.g. 1 ml dexamethason (Oradexon®, 1 ampoule of 1 ml containing 5 mg/ml)

- Administer oxygen (approximately 5 litres/minute)

- After these actions, have the patient transported to a hospital as soon as possible. Monitor the patient's heart rate and respiration continuously

corticosteroid must be injected. The administration of oxygen is recommended, and the patient must be transferred to the emergency department of a hospital as quickly as possible (Table 10.2).

Glottic oedema requires the same treatment. As long as any respiration is present, it is recommended to have the patient breath oxygen. In the case of a complete airway obstruction, an emergency intubation or tracheotomy is a last resort. Mild hypersensitivity reactions such as urticaria or itching do not *per se* require treatment; if necessary, oral administration of an antihistamine will suffice.

10.6.4 Strategy for suspected allergy

Since renewed exposure to an allergen can induce serious symptoms, especially in an immediate hypersensitivity reaction, treatment is aimed at preventing re-exposure of the patient to the same compound. However, one must realise that most unwanted reactions that patients attribute to an allergy are normal physiological reactions during stressful situations, psychogenic reactions or the result of a failed injection technique. Moreover, allergic reactions can also be induced by latex gloves or dental materials and erroneously be attributed to the administered local anaesthetic.

To investigate the possible cause of an allergic reaction after the administration of local anaesthesia, the detailed recording of information such as use of medication, the time frame of the reaction, previous reactions and current symptoms is an important starting point. All dental materials used during treatment should also be documented carefully.

Patients can be referred to an allergologist or dermatologist for further investigation. To determine whether a patient has a delayed hypersensitivity, the medical specialist will apply the suspected components of the anaesthetic separately on the skin (of the back). After 48 or 72 hours, the skin at these locations is inspected for a reaction. Patch tests are fairly reliable at demonstrating a delayed hypersensitivity reaction to a local anaesthetic.

To prove an immediate hypersensitivity reaction, intracutaneous tests can be used. Minimum amounts of the suspected anaesthetic or preservative are introduced into the skin, and subsequently a skin reaction will be looked for. These skin tests are not completely reliable. Therefore, sometimes a so-called provocation test is performed, during which the patient is deliberately exposed to the suspected local anaesthetic. Considering the risk of an anaphylactic reaction, these provocation tests are not without danger and may only be performed in a hospital. However, it seems more practical to perform a provocation test with the local anaesthetic that is considered as an alternative. The chance of a reaction is smaller and when the test is negative, this provides a safe alternative.

In a patient with a proved allergy to an amide type of anaesthetic, cross reactivity can make it difficult to find an alternative amide anaesthetic. In this case, one has to divert sometimes to an anaesthetic of the ester type. Fortunately, allergies to amide anaesthetics are very rare.

10.7 Prevention of side effects

A good explanation and fear-reducing treatment may prevent psychogenic reactions, the most common side effects, to a large extent. A medical history is essential to identify patients with an increased risk of side effects. In addition, it will identify medication that could interfere with the local anaesthetic.

Never administer more anaesthetic than absolutely necessary, using the lowest concentration of vasoconstrictor possible. During the entire dental treatment session, all cartridges used should remain on the worktop so that the total dose of anaesthetic administered can be calculated at any time. This avoids exceeding the maximum dose of anaesthetic during repeat injections during the treatment session. The risk of intravascular injection of (a part of) the local anaesthetic can be minimised by always aspirating before the injection. During the injection, the patient should be observed continuously and should be asked how he or she feels. In this way, undesired reactions will be noticed early. Never leave a patient unobserved after anaesthesia has been administered (Box 10.5).

Box 10.5 Some general preventive measures with regard to the use of local anaesthetics

- Take a medical history beforehand.
- Reassure the patient and give accurate information.
- Never use more anaesthetic than absolutely necessary.
- Use the lowest concentration vasoconstrictor possible.
- Place the patient in a half-seated to horizontal position.
- Aspirate.
- Inject slowly.
- Observe any reaction of the patient during the injection.
- Have a medical emergency kit with medication available.

When unwanted reactions occur during the injection of an anaesthetic, one refrains of course from further administration. Finally, the dental practice should have a medical emergency kit with medication and materials to provide adequate help in acute medical situations. This emergency kit should be inspected and updated regularly.

Patients at risk

H.S. Brand and J.F.M. Fennis

Dentists are increasingly confronted with medically compromised patients. In this chapter, systemic diseases will be discussed that are associated with a (theoretically) increased risk of side effects during the administration of local anaesthetics (Table 11.1).

11.1 Introduction

For the prevention of side effects of local anaesthesia it is important to identify patients with increased risk before administration. By taking a structured medical history, preferably written, the dentist usually can retrieve relevant information about the general health of the patient. It will also identify any medication that could interfere with the local anaesthetic.

When the patient reports a disease or condition that may interact with the administration of local anaesthetics, consultation with the patient's physician is advisable and sometimes necessary. To obtain this medical information from a general physician or medical specialist, explicit permission of the patient is required, preferably in written form.

11.2 Cardiovascular disease

Local anaesthetics reduce the contraction strength of the heart. Therefore, one has to consider the risk that latent heart failure may manifest itself during the administration of a local anaesthetic. In addition, liver perfusion is reduced in heart failure, which increases the half-life of amide-type anaesthetics and the risk of overdose. Since the transmission of action potentials in the heart is delayed under the influence of local anaesthetics, one also should consider – at least theoretically – the development of an atrioventricular block, which results in an abnormally slow heart rhythm accompanied by dizziness or loss of consciousness.

An increased adrenaline concentration in the blood results in an increased workload of the heart. In patients with ischaemic heart disease this will increase the oxygen deficit of the heart muscle, which may

Table 11.1	Recommendations for the use of local anaesthetics in medically compromised patients in general dental practice.		
	Local anaesthetic	*Vasoconstrictor*	*Other aspects*
Alcoholism	Reduce maximum dose		
Allergy towards			
– anaesthetic (documented)	Other type of anaesthetic (depending on allergy testing results)		Alternative: general anaesthesia
– antioxidant (bisulphite)		**Only adrenaline without bisulphite added**	**Bisulphite contraindicated** Alternative: felypressin containing anaesthetic
– latex			**Glass cartridges with rubber diaphragm contraindicated** Alternative: fill plastic syringe with anaesthetic
Anaemia	Reduce maximum dose of prilocaine		
Anaphylaxis: see allergy			
Angina pectoris			
– unstable	**Contraindicated**		
– other		Reduce adrenaline	
Anorexia nervosa	Reduce maximum dose		
Asthma			Preservatives discouraged
Basedow's disease: see hyperthyroidism			
Behavioural disorders			
– using medication		Reduce adrenaline	
Bleeding tendency: see haemorrhagic diathesis			
Bradycardia	Reduce maximum dose	Reduce adrenaline	
Bronchitis			
– chronic		Reduce adrenaline	Bilateral regional block anaesthesia discouraged
Cardiac rhythm abnormalities		Reduce adrenaline	

Table 11.1	Cont'd		
	Local anaesthetic	*Vasoconstrictor*	*Other aspects*
Cocaine – <24 h ago		**Adrenaline contraindicated**	
Coeliac disease	Reduce maximum dose		
COPD		Reduce adrenaline	Bilateral regional block anaesthesia discouraged
CVA – <1 year ago – >1 year ago		Reduce adrenaline	Consult patient's physician
Diabetes mellitus – poorly controlled		Reduce adrenaline	
Eczema – constitutional			Preservatives discouraged
Extreme fear (of needles, syringes, anaesthetic)			Alternatives: The Wand, general anaesthesia, premedication
G6PD-deficiency	Prilocaine discouraged		
Gastro-oesophageal reflux disease – using cimetidine	Reduce maximum dose		
Glaucoma		Reduce adrenaline	
Graves's disease: see hyperthyroidism			
Haemophilia – factor level <50%			Regional block anaesthesia discouraged
Haemorrhagic diathesis			Avoid regional blocks, if possible
Heart failure	Reduce maximum dose	Reduce adrenaline	
Heart infarction: see myocardial infarction			

Table 11.1	Cont'd		
	Local anaesthetic	*Vasoconstrictor*	*Other aspects*
Heart valve defects (including valve replacements)			Intraligamentary injection discouraged
Hepatitis	Reduce maximum dose		If necessary, use ester-type anaesthetic
Huntington's disease – using medication		Reduce adrenaline	
Hypertension		Reduce adrenaline	
Hyperthyroidism – uncontrolled		**Adrenaline contraindicated**	Postpone treatment
Hypoproteinaemia	Reduce maximum dose		
Hypothyroidism	Reduce maximum dose		
Ischaemic heart disease	Reduce maximum dose	Reduce adrenaline	
Kidney insufficiency	Reduce maximum dose		
Leukaemia – with increased bleeding tendency			Regional block anaesthesia discouraged
Liver cirrhosis	Reduce maximum dose		If necessary, use ester-type anaesthetic
Lung emphysema		Reduce adrenaline	Bilateral regional block anaesthesia discouraged
Malnutrition	Reduce maximum dose		
Marijuana – recent use			Adrenaline discouraged
Myasthenia gravis		Reduce adrenaline	
Myocardial infarction – < 6 weeks ago – > 6 weeks ago	**Contraindicated** Reduce maximum dose	Reduce adrenaline	Postpone treatment
Old age	Reduce maximum dose	Reduce adrenaline	
Oral antithrombotics: see haemorrhagic diathesis			

Table 11.1	Cont'd			
	Local anaesthetic	*Vasoconstrictor*	*Other aspects*	
Osteopetrosis		Reduce adrenaline		
Parkinson's disease – using medication		Reduce adrenaline		
Peptic ulcer – using cimetidine or proton pump inhibitor	Reduce maximum dose			
Pheochromocytoma		**Adrenaline contraindicated**		
Porphyria	Lidocaine and mepivacaine discouraged			
Pregnancy	Bupivacaïne discouraged; another anaesthetic with high degree of protein binding first choice; reduce maximum dose	Felypressin discouraged; reduce adrenaline	If possible postpone treatment	
Psychiatric disorders – using medication		Reduce adrenaline		
Radiotherapy – of head and neck area		Reduce vasoconstrictors		
Short bowel syndrome	Reduce maximum dose			
Sickle cell anaemia	Reduce maximum dose of prilocaine	Reduce adrenaline		
Spasticity			Injection needles in mouth discouraged. Alternative: inhalation sedation or general anaesthesia	
Systemic lupus erythematosus – advanced disease	Reduce maximum dose			
Thrombocytopenia – platelets < 50,000/mm^3			Avoid regional blocks, if possible	
von Willebrand's disease			Avoid regional blocks, if possible	

Reduce maximum dose = during one treatment session no more than 25–50% of the maximum recommended dose of the anaesthetic should be used.

Reduce adrenaline = during one treatment session the total amount of adrenaline should be restricted to a maximum of 0.04 mg for adults (= 4 ml adrenaline 1:100,000 or 8 ml adrenaline 1:200,000).

provoke an attack of angina pectoris or even a myocardial infarction. It is recommended that dental treatment, when necessary, is performed at least 6 weeks after a myocardial infarction. Furthermore, epinephrine can lead to heart rhythm disturbances.

Because pain during dental treatment induces a substantial increase in the release of adrenaline from the renal medulla, adequate anaesthesia is essential in patients with ischaemic heart diseases. According to the American Heart Association, use of adrenaline as vasoconstrictor is justified in a dilution of 1:100,000 or 1:200,000 and the total amount of adrenaline should be restricted to 0.04 mg for adults (= 4 ml anaesthetic solution with adrenaline 1:100,000 or 8 ml with 1:200,000), though this also depends on the weight of the patient. Of course, one should always aspire to minimise the risk of intravascular injection of adrenaline. A possible alternative for adrenaline is the use of prilocaine with the vasoconstrictor felypressin, which has no or only limited cardiac effects.

Patients with structural heart defects and/or prosthetic heart valves have an increased risk of developing infective endocarditis, an infection of the endothelium that covers the inside surface of the heart and the heart valves. Since most injections in the oral cavity do not induce a substantial bacteraemia, prophylactic use of an antibiotic is in general not necessary. However, endocarditis prophylaxis may be indicated for the subsequent dental procedure.

Intraligamentary anaesthesia may introduce considerable numbers of bacteria into the bloodstream. This injection technique should be avoided in patients at risk of infective endocarditis, unless antibiotic prophylaxis is already indicated for following invasive dental procedures.

11.3   Hypertension

The stress associated with the administration of a local anaesthetic induces an increase in blood pressure, both in healthy individuals and in patients with hypertension. Therefore, the severity of the hypertension must be determined before the administration of a local anaesthetic. One can ask the hypertensive patient whether his or her blood pressure has been measured recently and, if so, which values were determined at that moment. Dentists can also measure the patient's blood pressure themselves.

Patients with a systolic blood pressure exceeding 200 mmHg and/or a diastolic value over 115 mmHg should only receive dental treatment when their blood pressure has been medically treated. When the hypertensive patient has a systolic blood pressure between 160 and 200 mmHg or a diastolic pressure between 105 and 115 mmHg *and* the patient is currently under medical treatment, most dental treatment can be performed. Fear of the injection may induce a further increase in blood pressure. It is important to create an open atmosphere, where the patient feels free to discuss possible concerns about the intended injection and the dentist takes these into consideration.

Pain during dental treatment will also lead in hypertensive patients to a substantial release of adrenaline from the adrenal medulla, with a considerable increase in blood pressure. On the other hand, the use of large amounts of anaesthetic with adrenaline as vasoconstrictor or an accidental intravascular injection will raise the blood pressure too. Therefore it is recommended to use adrenaline in hypertensive patients only in a dilution of 1:100,000 or 1:200,000, and to restrict the total amount of adrenaline to 0.04 mg for adults (= 4 ml anaesthetic solution with adrenaline 1:100,000 or 8 ml with 1:200,000). Especially in this group of patients, one always has to aspirate *before* the injection of the local anaesthetic. One could also consider the use of local anaesthetics with felypressin as vasoconstrictor, as in patients with severe heart failure.

11.4 Cerebrovascular accident

Whether local anaesthetics can be used in patients with a cerebral infarction or bleeding depends on the length of time since the cerebrovascular accident (CVA) occurred and the current presence of certain risk factors. CVA patients currently suffering from transient ischaemic attacks (TIAs) should not receive elective dental care and consequently not receive local anaesthesia. With other CVA patients, the patient's physician should be consulted if the CVA occurred less than 1 year ago. In patients where the CVA occurred more than 1 year ago, a local anaesthetic may be used with a limited amount of adrenaline as vasoconstrictor (0.04 mg for adults).

11.5 Increased bleeding tendency

An increased bleeding tendency ('haemorrhagic diathesis') is usually caused by medication or a congenital disorder. To prevent excessive blood clotting, two types of drugs are used (antithrombotics): platelet aggregation inhibitors, of which the most important are acetylsalicylic acid (Aspirin®), carbasalate calcium (Ascal®) and clopidogrel bisulphate (Plavix®); and the coumarin derivatives acenocoumarol (Sintrom®) and phenprocoumon (Marcoumar®), which prevent the formation of a fibrin clot.

In patients using oral antithrombotics, the passage of an injection needle through tissues is associated with the risk of a large haematoma. Also in patients with an hereditary bleeding disorder, such as haemophilia, an extensive injection haematoma can develop. A severe bleeding in the pharyngeal tissues after mandibular block anaesthesia may cause an obstruction of the airway, which may even become life-threatening.

In patients with haemophilia, regional block anaesthesia should only be used if the concentration clotting factor is higher than 50% of the normal level. For patients using coumarin derivatives, an international normalised ratio (INR) below 3.5 to 4.0 can be used as a guideline.

A possible alternative is to use infiltration anaesthesia or intraligamentary anaesthesia in these patients, since these injection techniques are not associated with significant haematoma formation. In consultation with the haematologist, the anticoagulant level of patients treated with coumarin derivatives can temporarily be reduced by the administration of vitamin K. Another possibility is the use of antifibrinolytic therapy, such as the administration of tranexamic acid (Cyklokapron®).

11.6 Liver diseases

Patients with a severely impaired liver function, for example as a result of hepatitis or liver cirrhosis, are usually very ill. When administration of a local anaesthetic is indicated in these patients, one has to consider the reduced metabolism of amide-type anaesthetics in the liver and the increased risk of overdose. The reduced synthesis of albumin by the impaired liver decreases the protein binding of anaesthetics, further increasing the risk of overdose. In consultation with the patient's physician, one should aim for the lowest possible dose. The possible use of an ester-type anaesthetic, which is metabolised in plasma, can be considered (see Section 3.3.7).

11.7 Diabetes mellitus

Adrenaline has an antagonistic effect on insulin. Consequently, the administration of an anaesthetic with adrenaline as vasoconstrictor could potentially deregulate the blood glucose level of patients with diabetes mellitus. However, the dental treatment performed under local anaesthesia can interfere with the normal eating pattern, which usually affects the blood glucose level much more than the limited amount of adrenaline administered.

Only in insulin-dependent diabetics with poorly controlled blood glucose levels should the use of adrenaline as vasoconstrictor be reduced. Therefore, before administration of a local anaesthetic the dentist should verify the regulation of the diabetes. Nowadays, many patients with diabetes have a portable glucose meter that enables them to measure their own blood glucose level at any moment.

11.8 Hyperthyroidism

Thyroid hormone has a direct effect on the myocardium. As a result, increases in both heart rate and blood pressure are observed in patients with hyperthyroidism. These patients may also show unpredictable reactions after the administration of medication (idiosyncrasy). Thus, in patients with untreated hyperthyroidism, administration of a local anaesthetic may cause a thyrotoxic crisis. Elective dental treatment should be postponed until treatment of the hyperthyroidy is initiated. If local anaesthesia with a vasoconstrictor is unavoidable, felypressin is safer than adrenaline.

11.9 Hypoproteinaemia

In patients with hypoproteinaemia, toxic effects are observed at lower doses with those local anaesthetics with a high degree of binding to plasma proteins. Therefore, toxic levels will be reached more rapidly with articaine, which has a greater degree of protein binding than lidocaine and prilocaine. Medical conditions that may decrease plasma protein levels are anorexia nervosa, liver cirrhosis, chronic inflammatory bowel disease and nephrotic syndrome (leakage of protein from the kidneys to the urine). In these patients, one should keep the dose of the local anaesthetic as low as possible.

11.10 Pregnancy

The administration of a local anaesthetic with a vasoconstrictor may pose a risk for both the unborn child and the expectant mother. Current data indicate that articaine, lidocaine and mepivacaine can be used without danger to the foetus. Articaine seems the anaesthetic of choice: it has the greatest binding to plasma proteins, which will minimise transfer across the placenta to the foetus. On the other hand, prilocaine is able to induce methaemoglobinaemia in the foetus and should therefore be avoided (Box 11.1).

Felypressin is related to the hormone oxytocin, which induces uterine contractions during delivery. Therefore, this vasoconstrictor should be avoided during pregnancy. The amount of adrenaline should be restricted as this vasoconstrictor also has effects on the uterus. On the

---

Box 11.1 Methaemoglobinaemia

In erythrocytes, haemoglobin is normally present in the reduced state (Fe^{2+}). This reduced form is spontaneously gradually oxidised to the ferric form (Fe^{3+}), which results in the formation of methaemoglobin that is not able to carry oxygen. Under normal conditions, the level of methaemoglobin is limited to approximately 1% of the total amount of haemoglobin.

A degradation product of prilocaine, ortho-toluidine, can increase the level of methaemoglobin substantially, thereby causing hypoxia. In healthy adults, however, methaemoglobinaemia will only develop after the administration of high doses of prilocaine (400–600 mg). Treatment consists of intravenous administration of methylene blue.

other hand, pain during dental treatment should be prevented to avoid endogenous production of adrenaline.

Renal function may be reduced during pregnancy, resulting in an increased plasma concentration of the local anaesthetic and an increased risk of overdose for the expectant mother. This has been reported especially with bupivacaine.

Pregnancy is not an absolute contraindication for the administration of a local anaesthetic, but in many cases it will be possible to postpone dental treatment until after childbirth and even beyond breastfeeding. If dental treatment is required during pregnancy, it is best performed during the second trimester using not more than two to three cartridges of local anaesthetic.

11.11   Use of medication

In general, many drugs bind to plasma proteins and thereby compete with local anaesthetics that also bind to plasma proteins. This may lead to a reduction in the number of binding places available for local anaesthetics, increasing the free plasma levels and thus the toxicity of local anaesthetics. In addition, with some drugs more specific interactions with local anaesthetics have been described.

The action of *cell membrane stabilising medication*, such as phenytoin (Diphantoine®, Epanutin®), is potentiated by local anaesthetics and thereby could induce a cardiac toxic effect. Concomitant administration of a local anaesthetic and an *anti-arrhythmic agent* such as quinidine can enhance the effect on the atrioventricular conduction in the heart.

Sedatives, such as diazepam (Valium®, Stesolid®), increase the toxic effect of local anaesthetics. This dose-dependent effect seems to be mutual: the local anaesthetic intensifies the sedation.

Sulphonamides (e.g. Sulfadiazine®) affect the metabolism of prilocaine, which increases the risk of developing methaemoglobinaemia (Box 11.1). The histamine H_2-receptor antagonist *cimetidine*, used in the treatment of peptic ulcer and reflux disease, delays the degradation of lidocaine, leading to somewhat elevated plasma levels of this anaesthetic.

β-blockers interact with liver enzymes that metabolise amide-type anaesthetics. Since β-blockers also reduce the hepatic blood flow, this will result in an increased plasma concentration of the anaesthetic. Moreover, in cardiovascular patients treated with non-selective β-blockers (carvedilol, labetalol, oxprenolol, pindolol, propanolol and sotalol), adrenaline may lead to hypertension. In these patients, the blockade of the $β_2$-receptors prevents the vasodilatation in skeletal muscles that compensates the α-adrenergic vasoconstriction. This risk does not occur with selective β-blockers (atenolol, betaxolol, bisoprolol, celiprolol, esmolol, metoprolol and nebivolol).

Tricyclic antidepressants (e.g. amitriptyline, clomipramine) inhibit the re-uptake of adrenaline into nerve cells, which increases the concentration at the site of the receptor. Consequently, tricyclic antidepressants can potentially potentiate the cardiovascular effects of adrenaline. Therefore, in these patients the use of adrenaline as vasoconstrictor is discouraged. Other antidepressants, the so-called *monoamine oxidase inhibitors* (MAO inhibitors, e.g. phenelzine), inhibit the degradation of adrenaline in the central nervous system so that simultaneous use of adrenaline likewise increases the risk of a hypertensive reaction.

Phenothiazines (antipsychotics, e.g. chlorpromazine and perphenazine) block the α-adrenergic receptors. In these patients, administration of adrenaline may lead to a serious fall in blood pressure: the α-adrenergic vasoconstriction cannot occur, yet the β_2-adrenergic vasodilatation will take place. Therefore adrenaline should not be used as vasoconstrictor in patients using phenothiazines.

One also has to be careful with patients using *nose drops*. Nose drops sometimes contain the sympathicomimetic compound phenylephrine, causing unexpected strong effects of adrenaline. *Cocaine* and derivates like 'crack' are sympathicomimetics too. Therefore adrenaline is contraindicated as vasoconstrictor for individuals who have recently used cocaine.

Patients treated with corticosteroids for a long time may need an additional dose of corticosteroids during more extensive dental treatment ('stress-protocol'). This is not required for the administration of a local anaesthetic, but the necessity depends on the extension of the subsequent dental treatment or oral and maxillofacial surgery.

12 Legal aspects of local anaesthesia

W.G. Brands

The dentist should consider the possibility that, in certain cases, he/she may be asked to justify giving or permitting the application of local anaesthesia before a court. Verdicts, and the laws on which they are based, differ from country to country and often even differ within a country, e.g. within the United States, Canada and Australia. It is necessary to keep in mind that a dentist is only subject to the law of the country, province or state in which he/she is currently practising. Despite this variance, there are many similarities between the various jurisdictions. Therefore, comments on the legal aspects of the use of local anaesthetics in dentistry often have international value.

A dentist may be summoned before various judges, each of whom will consider the case according to his or her own criteria. For this reason, first the different courts that may judge a dentist's case are described in this chapter. Subsequently, the competency of the dentist and co-workers with regard to the administration of local anaesthesia is discussed. Following this, several cases illustrate the kind of legal problems a dentist may be confronted with after applying local anaesthesia and the circumstances under which the dentist may be held to account. Finally, suggestions are given of how to reduce the risk of juridical problems after the administration of local anaesthesia.

12.1 Judges and courts

If a patient believes he or she has been treated unjustly by his/her dentist, the patient may file a formal complaint to various courts. The patient's choice of the different courts will usually be influenced by two considerations:
- How simple and expensive is the legal procedure?
- What will I gain from the procedure?

Usually, the complainant hopes that the accused dentist will receive a form of punishment or caution, and that the damage suffered will be compensated. Depending on his/her aim, the patient may approach the following judges or courts:

1 *The disciplinary board.* Applying to this board is generally a free procedure. The board considers whether disciplinary measures should be imposed on the dentist, and these measures may vary from a caution to prohibiting the dentist from practising. For the dentist, this legal proceeding is very unpleasant, not only because of the potential punitive measures, but also because of the publicity. Many dental boards publish the names of the involved dentists online, especially in cases of a suspension or a permanent prohibition to practise dentistry. Some boards even provide complete case files, including the dentist's full name, for public inspection. Such boards include the General Dental Council in Great Britain (http://www.gdc-uk.org) and disciplinary councils in Colorado (USA) (http://www.dora.state.co.us/DENTAL/), New Zealand (http://www.dcnz.org.nz/) and Victoria (Australia) (http://www.dentprac.vic.gov.au/decisions.asp).

2 *The criminal court.* By submitting a complaint, the patient starts a procedure which may eventually lead to the prosecution of the dentist according to the criminal law. Because criminal law is regarded as an utmost serious measure, dentists rarely are confronted with the criminal court. However, if a patient should die after administration of local anaesthesia, a criminal law procedure is nowadays likely. For the average law-abiding dentist, a criminal law procedure and certainly a consequent prison sentence will be quite a traumatic experience. In the United States and countries within the Commonwealth, a disciplinary procedure will be started automatically against dentists who are convicted according to criminal law, often without the involvement of the respective patient.

3 *The civil law court.* If a patient has suffered damage for which the dentist is responsible, the patient may summon the dentist before a civil law court. The procedure usually follows in writing. Though the civil judge gives a verdict concerning the damages of the patient, this verdict in most cases does not include any penalty. A disadvantage for the dentist is that a civil law case is often very expensive. The compensation to be paid can reach incredible proportions, especially in the United States. This usually concerns cases where the dentist's reckless treatment has led to permanent medical damage to the patient. In the United States, in such cases so-called punitive damages may be imposed. In countries of the Commonwealth this compensation is called an exemplary damage award. The following case from New Zealand demonstrates that there are very strict grounds upon which punitive damage is awarded.

Case: Punitive damage in dentistry
(NZCA 215, 1999, New Zealand)

During endodontic treatment, a part of an endodontic instrument remained in the patient's root canal. The patient claimed she suffered from repeated inflammation and pain. Allegations relate to the original treatment and failure to notice that the instrument had fractured, with part remaining in the tooth, the failure to discover or disclose the presence of the fragment and to take steps to relieve the pain, and generally acting in a high-handed manner by never admitting the negligent conduct or offering assistance. It is alleged that these matters were aggravated by oppressive tactics adopted by the dentist after notice had been given of the intention to take proceedings. The claim was for exemplary damages of NZ $250,000.

The court stated about the exemplary damages: "The indications from the evidence presently available consist more with the dentist not having discovered the fragment. Mrs X confirmed that this is the allegation. It may be a case of negligence but not of a kind that would attract exemplary damages. Failure by a medical or dental caregiver to investigate a suspected cause of persistent pain or discomfort, though negligent, would be likely to attract an award of exemplary damages only where the dentist is shown to have had improper motive, reckless disregard for the patient's health or safety, or some special flagrancy reflecting the type of conduct that amounts to an affront to the community. It is not enough to simply allege that the caregiver is high-handed. This case involves allegations of negligence that may be possible to prove but it is not sufficient to be one of those rare cases in which exemplary damages might be awarded."

In a study by Cohen (2005) it appeared that the median amount for punitive damage was US $187,000, with a peak of $75 million. Punitive damage is usually awarded in cases relating to general medical practice; very rarely is it awarded in dentistry cases.

One difference between disciplinary and criminal law on the one hand and civil law on the other hand is especially significant for dental practices where many treatments are delegated to an employee. The disciplinary and criminal courts are only interested in whether the dentist him/herself is to blame. The reproach may be that the dentist him/herself has been insufficiently cautious in the application of local anaesthesia, but also that he/she has delegated the application incorrectly. One can, however, also approach a civil law court if the dentist is not personally to blame, but rather one of his/her staff.

12.2   Competency to give local anaesthesia

The competencies of medical professionals are generally described in a law that governs the medical professions. A special law for dentistry, a Dental Practice act, is not uncommon. Often these laws are relatively general and are implemented following the guidelines of the dental boards or of the national dental practitioners' organisation.

12.2.1   General and local anaesthesia given by the dentist

In almost all countries, giving anaesthesia is considered a relatively hazardous procedure that may not be performed by just anyone. In some cases the law appears to regard anaesthesia as more dangerous than, for instance, an extraction. Article 139 A of the Dental Practitioners Registration Act (2001) in Queensland (Australia), for example, states that in an emergency an unqualified person may extract a tooth in the absence of a dentist but cannot give a local anaesthetic.

Usually a distinction is made between giving local anaesthesia and general anaesthesia. On the basis of the dentist's education, or in many states on the basis of his/her licence, a dentist is generally qualified to administer a local anaesthetic. An additional licence is usually required for giving general anaesthesia and special conditions are required for the dental practice. For example, the guidelines for giving general anaesthesia in Ontario (Canada) demand that the dentist has followed a course on narcosis and sedation which shows that he/she is capable of giving general anaesthesia. In some countries, such as the Netherlands, there is no obligation to obtain a separate certificate, but the dentist must demonstrate with a course diploma that he/she is skilled in giving (local) anaesthesia. In practice, the two systems do not differ greatly.

12.2.2   Local anaesthesia given by paramedics

Worldwide there are various paramedics active in dental practice. Because their titles and corresponding qualifications differ from country to country, this section will explore the main professionals involved: the dental assistant, the dental hygienist and the dental therapist.

The dental assistant has a relatively low level of dental education and in most countries is not qualified to give local anaesthesia. In some countries an exception is made with regard to the application of topical anaesthesia. In the state of Montana (USA), for example, a dental assistant may apply topical anaesthesia under the direct supervision of a dentist (Montana, Board of Dentistry rule 24.138.406). The Netherlands provides an exception to this point, since in this country a dental assistant is permitted to give local anaesthesia provided that a dentist has given the order, the assistant is competent and there is a form of supervision (Article 38 BIG). A Dutch dentist must be able to demonstrate that all conditions have been met. If this is not the case, both the assistant and the dentist may face a jail sentence. With such measures, the Dutch authorities try to prevent unqualified dental assistants from giving local anaesthesia.

The conditions under which *dental hygienists* may administer local anaesthetics vary widely internationally. In the Netherlands, a dental hygienist is qualified to give local anaesthesia for dental treatments, even in the absence of the dentist. In most other countries, a dental hygienist is only permitted to give local anaesthesia under supervision. If this requirement is not met, disciplinary measures will follow.

Some jurisdictions, such as Canadian and Australian provinces, also recognise the *dental therapist*. This assistant has more extensive qualifications than the dental hygienist, including being qualified to administer local anaesthesia.

Case: Unqualified application of a mandibular block
(South Carolina State Board of Dentistry, USA)

A dentist permitted his dental hygienist to give a mandibular block without the required supervision. In principle, this would result in a suspension of his licence for 5 years. He agreed with the dental board, however, that he would pay a fine of US $3000, follow a course in ethics and would redo his exam in jurisprudence. Furthermore, he would pay utmost attention that insufficiently qualified staff would no longer perform treatments in his practice.

12.3 Liability

There are only a few cases known where the administration of a local anaesthetic has led to a complaint or claim. In the following section, various situations will be discussed in which the administration of a local anaesthetic has led to legal proceedings. The reader must bear in mind that jurisprudence in one country does not automatically apply to dental practices in other countries. Nevertheless, the cases presented provide a reasonable overview of what a dentist may be blamed for by a patient if the administration of anaesthesia does not go according to plan.

12.3.1 A damaged nerve following anaesthesia: informed consent

Case: Nerve damage following a mandibular block
(Dental Board Utrecht, The Netherlands)

A patient retained a partly anaesthetised tongue following a mandibular block. The anaesthesia was given for soft tissue treatment. When asked, the dentist explained that the nerve had been touched during the anaesthesia, but that the symptoms would most likely disappear. However, the symptoms did not disappear and the patient pressed charges. The patient based his complaint on the fact that prior to the treatment the dentist had given insufficient information regarding the possible risks. The patient explained that loss of feeling in the tongue significantly hindered his eating and his social life. He also suffered from insomnia and headaches. The dental board judged that the dentist could not be blamed for pricking the lingual nerve and that there is a consensus within the profession that patients do not need to be informed of very rare risks. The charge was dismissed.

In the above-mentioned case the complaint was rejected because the risk of the particular complication was very small. According to the available literature the incidence of permanent damage to the lingual nerve as a result of anaesthesia varies between 1 in 26,000 to 1 in 800,000 (Pogrel *et al.*, 2003). If transient sensitivity disorders are included, the incidence increases to 1 in 2667 (van Dam and Bruers, 2004).

The dental board assumed in the above case that the dentist was not required to warn the patient on the basis of the risk being so small. The disciplinary court took as a starting point for their judgment the fact that the dentist was reasonable, competent and well-practising. In various countries, such as Great Britain, Canada, the Netherlands and some states of the USA, it counts not only whether or not a reasonable practising dentist should have warned the patient of this risk, but also whether or not a reasonable patient would have refused anaesthesia in the same situation if he/she had been sufficiently informed (Brands, 2006). In answer to the last question, the following factors will be of importance:
• What was the risk that the complication might occur?
• How would the situation have developed without treatment?
• Could other, less risky treatment methods have been employed? If so, what was the chance of success of such treatment?
• How serious was the complication?

The above requirements are interdependent. A sensible patient will take a relatively large risk for a life-saving operation. On the other hand, a patient will hardly accept any risk for cosmetic surgery. If we apply these principles to the question of whether a patient must be informed of certain risks of local anaesthesia, we must make the following considerations.

Damage to a nerve may be hardly invalidating or life-threatening, but it does cause particular discomfort. The risk of damage to a nerve as a result of the administration of local anaesthesia is, however, so small that a reasonable patient will easily agree to anaesthesia for necessary dental treatment.

The situation is different if the patient's health will not be damaged in any way when he or she refrains from treatment, for example if the treatment is required simply for cosmetic reasons. Imagine that the dentist from the case above had administered local anaesthesia to replace an amalgam restoration with a composite white filling for cosmetic reasons. In this case it is questionable whether a reasonable patient will regard the small risk as acceptable.

Finally, a reasonable patient would not have accepted any risks at all if less risky alternatives were available. In that case the question is why the dentist has not considered, for example, the use of intraligamental anaesthesia instead of mandibular block anaesthesia (Loomer and Perry, 2004). If an anaesthetic technique is available that reduces the chance of nerve damage, the dentist has a greater obligation to inform the patient sufficiently when he chooses the more risky injection technique.

When a dentist knows more about a patient, the reasonable patient becomes less abstract and the dentist may decide differently. For example, patients who have to speak a lot in their profession will be less willing to accept a permanently anaesthetised lip than someone who works with his or her hands. This means that, when giving anaesthesia, the dentist should warn a singer more readily and extensively of the risks of sensitivity disorders than, for example, a car mechanic.

Another question is whether informed consent for giving local anaesthesia should be obtained verbally or in writing. Legislation on this point varies widely, so that nothing much helpful can be said about it globally. Otherwise, the general consensus worldwide is that a dentist must be able to demonstrate the informed consent. Written permission by the patient can therefore also be very useful in jurisdictions where dentists are not obliged to obtain written informed consent. An American study has shown that dental specialists usually record written informed consent, while general dental practitioners obtain written informed consent less frequently (Orr and Curtis, 2005).

12.3.2   No anaesthesia given, faulty injection or insufficient anaesthesia

For children, anaesthesia can often be a necessity. A very far-reaching verdict was given by the Dentistry Examining Board of Wisconsin (USA) in the following case.

Case: Treatment of children without anaesthesia
(Wisconsin Court of Appeals 02-2218, USA)

A dentist treated dental caries in four children under the age of 3 years. He did not use anaesthesia, nor did he inform the parents of the options for the administration of anaesthesia. After charges had been pressed, the dental board determined that the treatment of two children had been substandard. The board reprimanded the dentist and limited his licence to the treatment of children over 14 years old. The board also obliged him to attend a course in pain control.

A similar verdict – though in a case involving an adult – was pronounced by the Professional Conduct Committee (PCC) of the General Dental Council (GDC) in Great Britain.

Case: Treatment of adults without anaesthesia
(Professional Conduct Committee, Great Britain)

A dentist began a root canal treatment. He did not perform a sensitivity test and started to drill without giving anaesthesia. The PCC judged that without a sensitivity test the dentist could not know whether the tooth was vital or not and therefore should not have performed the treatment without anaesthesia or without explanation to the patient that the treatment could be painful. In this case the PCC judged it necessary that permission from the patient should have been obtained before drilling without anaesthesia.

The above cases concerned not giving anaesthesia; it is clear that the option of anaesthesia must, in any case, be offered to the patient. If subsequently anaesthesia is given, the dentist must observe the patient's behaviour very well to ascertain whether anything is wrong.

Case: The patient indicates during the injection that something is wrong
(Professional Conduct Committee, Great Britain)

Charges were pressed against a dentist for several matters concerning practice and incorrect treatments. One of the charges concerned the administration of anaesthesia. In the first place, the dentist was blamed for giving anaesthesia without obtaining informed consent. During the administration of anaesthesia, the dentist perforated the nose floor and injected the anaesthetic into the nasal cavity. The charge was not only that the dentist had perforated the nose floor, but also that the dentist continued with the treatment when the patient indicated that something was wrong during the administration of anaesthesia.

The Conduct Committee concluded that the dentist's knowledge was lacking in a number of areas and that these flaws needed to be corrected.

The patient's behaviour may also be important once the actual treatment has commenced and the patient indicates that the anaesthesia is not working.

Case: The patient indicates that the anaesthesia is not working
(Disciplinary Court, the Netherlands)

A patient was receiving a number of dental implants, for which anaesthesia had been administered. The anaesthesia worked for about 40 minutes. Although the anaesthesia had lost its effect, the dentist continued with the treatment because it was not yet completely finished. The patient subsequently lodged a complaint against the dentist, partly because of the painful treatment. The disciplinary court judged concerning the anaesthesia that it had been perfectly possible to give an additional amount of anaesthetic and that the dentist had been wrong not to do so. Because the disciplinary court also doubted the necessity for the implants, the dentist was given a caution.

In this case, the administration of an additional amount of anaesthetic had been possible. There are also cases where a local anaesthetic that has been applied correctly is not sufficiently effective, for example in certain forms of pulpitis. In such cases it is particularly important to inform the patient correctly. If there is a moderate chance that the patient cannot be fully anaesthetised, it is reasonable to assume the patient may refuse to give permission. If a dentist cannot convince the patient that the treatment should nevertheless be performed, it must be postponed. There may also be cases where the patient thinks he or she feels something during the treatment. In this case the dentist should give additional anaesthesia. If this is not successful, the dentist must consider whether the treatment can be halted or whether a 'point of no return' has been passed. In the latter case, the dentist could proceed with the treatment until a moment is reached where the situation is stable again.

12.3.3 Application of anaesthesia and general medical complications: record-keeping

Local anaesthesia is usually administered with an injection. The dentist must appreciate that receiving an injection may be an uncomfortable event for many people. Therefore, some patients may attribute misunderstood, unexpected or inexplicable events to the giving of an anaesthetic. The following two cases demonstrate this.

Case: Miscarriage
(Louisiana Court of Appeal, no, 98 Ca 0361 C/W 98 Ca 0362, USA)

A female patient approached a dentist complaining of pain. The dentist found a small abscess on a tooth, but advised postponement of the treatment because the patient was pregnant. The pain persisted and the dentist decided on a root canal treatment. The patient was anaesthetised using Citanest. Twelve days later the patient had a miscarriage and blamed this on the administered local anaesthetic. Since the consulted expert stated that the administered dose was defensible for a woman in the second trimester of her pregnancy, the charge was dismissed.

In another example, a patient claimed there was a link between inexplicable pain symptoms and an allergy to the anaesthetic.

Case: Allergy
(Dental Board, 10 May 2001, the Netherlands)

A filling was placed in a patient's tooth under local anaesthesia. Later, pulpitis emerged and the molar was opened under local anaesthesia. After this, the patient returned once again, but this did not result in further treatment. According to the patient, the dentist could not do anything for him, whilst the dentist claimed this was because the patient had physical complaints and should first be tested for a possible allergy to dental materials – on the patient's record was written 'allergy-nutrition; no dent. restrict. Quickly short of breath.'

Finally, charges were pressed against the dentist for giving anaesthesia twice without establishing whether the patient was allergic to it. The complainant, father of the patient, suggested that the dentist had used the anaesthetic articaine. The complainant had deduced this from the fact that the patient had felt nothing during treatment by the accused dentist and that the patient had felt pain during treatment by another dentist under prilocaine in combination with laser acupuncture. The accused dentist claimed to have used prilocaine and the disciplinary court had no reason to doubt this. The disciplinary court deliberated that it was highly unlikely that an allergic reaction to the anaesthetic had occurred that had led to a pulpitis, and dismissed the charge.

Probably, the above case would have been judged in the same way in most other countries.

These cases show that good record-keeping is extremely important. Especially with special patients such as pregnant women, patients with an allergy or another systemic disorder, it is incredibly important to record in the file which anaesthetic has been used and what dosage has been given. It seems that the dentist in the allergy case had a narrow escape. The disciplinary court took for granted that the dentist had used prilocaine and not articaine. The dentist in this case was treated very generously. In the United States, however, several dentists have been sentenced because they did not record in their files the type and dosage of the anaesthetic, or a recent medical history.

In the above cases it was assumed that there was no connection between the local anaesthetic and the medical complaints. After administration of a local anaesthetic, however, medical problems may occur where a direct connection could be assumed between the anaesthesia and the problem.

Case: Overdose
(Colorado State Board of Dental Examiners, USA)

A dentist extracted seven primary teeth in a child. For the anaesthesia, he used one cartridge of Citanest Plain and three cartridges of Citanest Forte. During the treatment the child suffered convulsions which subsided after a while, but the child remained unconscious for some time. The Dental Board assumed that this temporary unconsciousness had been caused by the high dose of local anaesthetic. The maximum dose for a patient of this weight was 180.4 mg prilocaine, while the dentist had administered a total of 288 mg. Charges were pressed against the dentist and considered well-founded.

Aside from the anaesthetic, systemic complications may also arise from the added vasoconstrictor.

Case: Brain haemorrhage after local anaesthesia
(Washington supp court, 28 Wn App 50, USA)

A patient approached his dentist for a wisdom-tooth extraction. The previous day, the patient had suffered from such a severe headache it had felt like his head would explode. The patient was unaware that he was suffering from hypertension and this had never been diagnosed. At the dentist's office he completed a written medical history, after which the dentist gave him an adrenaline-containing local anaesthetic. After the extraction, the patient became unwell. The following day, his condition deteriorated and a brain haemorrhage or brain infarction was diagnosed. The patient became disabled and died some time later. The dentist was summoned, partly because he had not verified if the patient suffered from hypertension. An expert stated that neglecting to measure the patient's blood pressure went against good care practice in that region at that time. Furthermore, it was considered significant that a textbook warned against the use of adrenaline in patients with hypertension and that the dentist chose not to perform the rather simple blood pressure measurement. One of the judges, however, held the opinion (a concurring opinion) that the statement of the expert did not clarify whether in such cases a dentist should ask if a patient is suffering from hypertension or whether the dentist should measure the patient's blood pressure anyway.

From a dental perspective some questions can be raised concerning this case, for example whether there was a clear relation between the vasoconstrictor and the brain haemorrhage. Stress could also have played a role, such as in a similar case in Texas (Court of Appeals Fifth District of Texas, White v Presnall), or it may have been a case of an intravasal injection. One may also wonder whether the expert was perhaps discussing too much retrospectively, for almost all systemic complications after extractions can be avoided if the dentist not only takes an adequate medical history, but also consults the patient's general physician or specialist or performs a basic physical examination him- or herself. However, it is not likely that this can be expected of a well-practising dentist, since this would create an unworkable situation. What can be learnt from this case is that, when choosing the local anaesthetic and vasoconstrictor, the dentist should always realise the consequences of this choice for the respective patient. The choice of a specific anaesthetic must be based on a recent medical history that is recorded in the patient's file, if the dentist is wise.

12.3.4 Insufficient caution during injection

Occasionally a dentist may be charged for not having exercised enough caution while giving anaesthesia so that a needle breaks, or if he/she did not use a sterile needle.

Case: Assistant pricked first and then the patient
(Court of Special Appeals of Maryland, USA)

A child required a root canal treatment and an extraction. Because the child was wriggling, the dental assistant held the child steady. When giving the anaesthesia the dentist first inadvertently pricked the assistant and then used the same needle for the patient. The next day, the dentist asked the mother to have the child tested for hepatitis. According to the dentist, the patient was pricked first and then the assistant. The mother phoned the dental assistant who said the opposite had been the case. Eventually an article appeared in a local paper, which attracted the attention of the dental board. On the basis of this incident and other complaints, the dentist's licence was revoked.

Nowadays, local anaesthesia is administered with disposable needles and cartridges. Cases where a needle and cartridge are used for two different people are extremely rare. This does not alter the fact that a dentist should realise that mistakes can be made during the administration of local anaesthesia. For this reason, dentists should give serious consideration to how to minimise complaints about the use of local anaesthesia.

12.4 ▍ Avoiding legal problems in the use of local anaesthesia

Dentists can avoid many juridical problems by some preventative measures:

- The dentist must be aware of his or her duties, particularly the duty to provide information.
- Without adequate medical history, recorded on the patient's file, any defence will fail.
- If there is any doubt whether anaesthesia is possible and, if so, under which conditions it may be performed, it is sensible to consult the patient's general physician or an oral and maxillofacial surgeon.
- If a dentist consults colleagues or takes special precautionary measures, it is wise to note this in the patient's file.
- The burden of the treatment must be as low as possible, especially for medically compromised patients. This may mean that the treatment is performed in more than one session, but also that a treatment may be postponed.
- If the dentist is not obliged to record every use of anaesthesia in the file, it is advised that the dentist notes in the file when he or she finds it necessary to use another anaesthetic to the usual one.

If the country where the dentist works allows the delegation of the administration of anaesthesia, the following points should be considered:

- The dentist must be aware of the conditions under which this is permissible. Dentists must be convinced themselves that the person they delegate the anaesthesia to has the necessary skills.
- There must be a clear protocol for the administration of anaesthesia, especially to patients at risk, and the procedure in case of complications.
- It is advisable only to delegate if a dentist or doctor can be at the scene very quickly in case of complications. This is automatically the case in jurisdictions where supervision is a prerequisite. In that case the dentist is legally obliged to be at the scene.

Naturally, these guidelines cannot guarantee absolute protection from complaints concerning the use of anaesthesia. However, legal problems are hopefully reduced by them.

Further reading

Brands, W.G. (2006) The standard for the duty to inform patients about risks: from the responsible dentist to the reasonable patient. *British Dental Journal*, **201**, 207–210.

Cohen, T.H. (2005) *Punitive Damage Awards in Large Counties 2001*. US Department of Justice, NCJ 208445, March 2005.

van Dam, B. & Bruers, J. (2004) Permanent sensitivity disorders in patients. *Nederlands Tandartsenblad,* **59** (16), 36–37.

Loomer, P.M. & Perry, D.A. (2004) Computer-controlled delivery versus syringe delivery of local anesthetic injections for therapeutic scaling and root planing. *JADA,* **135**, 358–365.

Orr, D.L. & Curtis, W.J. (2005) Obtaining written informed consent for the administration of local anesthetic in dentistry. *JADA,* **136**, 1568–1570.

Pogrel, M.A., Schmidt, B.L., Sambajon, V. & Jordan R.C.K. (2003) Lingual nerve damage due to inferior alveolar nerve blocks. *JADA,* **134**, 195–198.

Index